CHALLENGE & CRISIS
IN MISSIONARY MEDICINE

CHALLENGE & CRISIS IN MISSIONARY MEDICINE

DAVID J. SEEL

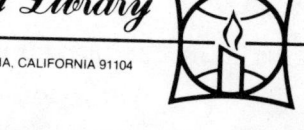

William Carey Library

1705 N. SIERRA BONITA AVE. • PASADENA, CALIFORNIA 91104

Library of Congress Cataloging in Publication Data

Seel, David John, 1925-
  Challenge and crisis in missionary medicine.

  Includes bibliographical references.
  1. Seel, David John, 1925-   2. Missionaries,
Medical--Korea--Biography. 3. Missions, Medical.
I. Title.
R722.32.S4A33   266'.025'0924   79-16015
ISBN 0-87808-172-0

Copyright © 1979 by David J. Seel

All rights reserved.

No part of this book may be used or reproduced in any manner whatsoever without written permission, except in the case of brief quotations embodied in critical articles and reviews.

Published by the William Carey Library
1705 N. Sierra Bonita Avenue
Pasadena, California 91104
Telephone (213) 798-0819

In accord with some of the most recent thinking of the academic press, the William Carey Library is pleased to present this scholarly book which has been prepared from an author-edited and author-prepared camera ready copy.

PRINTED IN THE UNITED STATES OF AMERICA

Contents

Foreword — *vii*
Preface — *ix*

Chapter

1. The Dilemma — 1
2. Why a Christian Hospital? — 15
3. A Philosophy of Medical Mission — 27
4. The Truth Beyond Faith and Science — 43
5. A Repository for the Value of the Individual — 59
6. Witness to the Preeminence of Christ — 75
7. The Corporate Life-Style of Love — 87
8. "Does Anyone Know I'm Here?" — 97

Chapter

9	Critical Opinions	111
10	Paraklesis	125

Notes   141

Foreword

How obvious it appears! Medicine and missions belong together like a shoe and foot. Jesus himself placed the two together. As he traveled Palestine teaching and preaching, he healed all kinds of diseases. Lepers came cringing into his presence and ran away clean. Blind men stumbled close to him left seeing. Deaf people heard his voice. James, Jesus' half brother, spelled out the responsibilities for curing souls and bodies. "Is any among you sick? Let him summon the elders of the congregation and let them pray over him anointing him with oil in the name of the Lord." Ministry and medicine -- prayer and oil -- make good partners. What God joined together should not be separated.

How simple it seems -- especially for us today. Christ's men and women in earlier times struggled along with limited remedies, but we have gotten far beyond a rubdown with oil. Modern technology treats diseases we did not even know existed a hundred years ago. Now, as we take the gospel to cultures primitive compared to our own, we offer also the advantages of western medicine. No longer need we touch the lepers, the blind, the fereish, the lame. Instead we can erect hospitals, put in the machines, process the sick, and heal them.

How demonic it becomes. Developing nations not only get the best of modern medicine but the worst. We know that technology is not an undiluted benefit. Giant machines turn American hospitals into expensive healing factories. A patient arrives at the admitting desk as a person, then a specialist turns her into a problem -- the gall bladder case in Room 331. Doctors at the foot of the bed read the charts and call for the tests.

Christians may naively equate bringing health to the nations with exporting western technology and technicians to other countries in the name of God. Jesus can be lost in his own hospital. Myriads of pressures, subtle and obvious, shove Christ out of the institution his followers have built. Medicine remains but ministry disappears.

That, in essence, stands as the *Challenge and Crisis in Missionary Medicine*, and that explains why this is an important book. Dr. David Seel serves Christ as a surgeon in Korea, but his book and the issues he deals with are as wide as the world. In any ministry, how easily the shoe tells the foot how to grow. Worse still, how much effort can be expended making better, more elaborate shoes for a foot that has been amputated.

Haddon W. Robinson
General Director
Christian Medical Society

Preface

Many hands and hearts participated in the preparation of this book. I have drawn from experience and dialogue in the corporate life of our hospital. In so doing I have not mentioned names of team members whose ideas and convictions have undoubtedly contributed to the elaboration of my own thinking. I have sought to give credit to all whose writings have helped in the development of the thesis here presented.

It is my hope that the challenges and the dilemmas of Christian medical ministry will be seen in their proper worldwide context. Doubtless more widely traveled participants in this ministry could bring broader insights from medical mission and service in other parts of the world. My commitments to the work in Korea preclude such an overview. Yet I am convinced that discerning how we may faithfully follow Christ in compassionate ministry is a matter which requires the attention of God's people everywhere.

I am particularly grateful to Mr. Charles C. Parvin, of the Chicago Tribune, who spent a month with us in Korea reviewing the manuscript, for many helpful editorial criticisms and improvements. I remain ever grateful for my wife's encouragement and for her stenographic skills.

This book is dedicated to all who have been stirred by the love of Christ, and have become participants in his paraklesis.

David John Seel, M.D., FACS

1

I tended him. God healed him.

> Ambroise Pare,[1]
> Military Surgeon
> 1510 - 1590

Our profession is a priestly ministry. I should like to see the Church consecrating doctors just as it ordains its ministers. This would be in conformity with the gospel. It is this conviction which makes us give ourselves with our hearts and minds and souls to our vocation. . .

> Paul Tournier, M.D.[2]

The Dilemma

The annals of Christian medicine are filled with heroes: Vanderkemp, Livingstone, Strangway and Schweitzer in Africa; Scudder in India; Parker and Cochrane in China; Allen and Avison in Korea. Most of them began alone in simple dispensaries. Most recognized the need for training national medical leaders; a few established hospitals which continue until this day. Occasionally missionary physicians have been in a position to make scientific breakthroughs in discovering the cause of a ravaging illness or in devising an effective treatment.

These pioneers were neither eloquent apologists for the Christian faith nor sophisticated medical specialists even by the standards of their day. Yet they perceived, and obeyed, a fundamental truth of Christian doctrine: that God is concerned with human pain and affliction and that any proclamation of the Christian gospel which neglects the alleviation of human suffering is not only incomplete but distorted and unfair to Jesus Christ. This truth consumed them. They accepted the

The Dilemma

agony of involvement, the fevers, the leeches, the diarrhea, the physical abuse, the ridicule, even solitary death in remote corners of the globe. Are there today those who could sincerely plead before their Creator the words of David Livingstone? "Send me anywhere, only go with me. Lay any burden on me, only sustain me. Sever any tie but the tie that binds me to Thy Service and to Thy Heart!"(3)

In the history of medical missions on the Korean peninsula, one man's brief but remarkable contribution illustrates the heroic dedication of those obsessed with the gospel of Christian mercy. He was Dr. Wiley Forsythe, a native of Mercer County, Kentucky, and a graduate of the Hospital College of Medicine, in Louisville. At the age of 30 he was appointed to serve in Jeonju (Chonju) in 1904. Within a year he had made remarkable record in medical witness. In March 1905 he was called to the country to treat a man of a prominent family who had been injured by bandits. As the missions historian, George T. Brown, chronicled the incident,

> after doing what he could for the patient, he went to sleep in the injured man's home, as it was too late to return that night. During the night the robbers returned. Mistaking Dr. Forsythe's foreign clothing for those of a policeman, they cut him badly with their knives and swords, leaving several gashes about his head and neck. . . He was first cared for by the Korean mistress of the home in which he was staying, and later

> faithful friends carried him tenderly back to Chonju where he received further treatment. But the badly lacerated wounds on his ear and head did not heal properly, and he had to return to the States for recuperation.(4)

He returned to Korea in 1908 to open new work in the southwestern port city of Mokpo. His zeal was such that he would take to the streets of the city "dispensing gospel tracts with one hand and medicines with the other." (5) Early in the Spring of 1909 Dr. Clement Owen, a medical and evangelistic missionary, lay dying of pneumonia at the hospital in Kwangju. Dr. R. M. Wilson, alarmed, sent for Dr. Forsythe for consultation. He started out from Mokpo by hoseback, not knowing that Dr. Owen had already died. Thirteen miles from Kwangju he encountered, by the side of the road, a woman with far-advanced leprosy, ragged and filthy. He lifted her to his saddle and led the horse on foot the remaining distance into the city. His intention to have her admitted to the hospital was thwarted when an outcry immediately arose from other patients, who did not want to be contaminated, so a makeshift shelter was arranged for her in an abandoned brick kiln, used in the hospital's construction. Mrs. Owen contributed her late husband's country bedding roll. Dr. Forsythe, grasping the arm of the woman, "loathsome from disease, filth, and long neglect,. . . her hair uncombed perhaps for months,. . . her feet and hands swollen and covered with sores," (6) helped her over the bricks and stones into her new quarters, as though escorting his own mother. She lived but two weeks, but

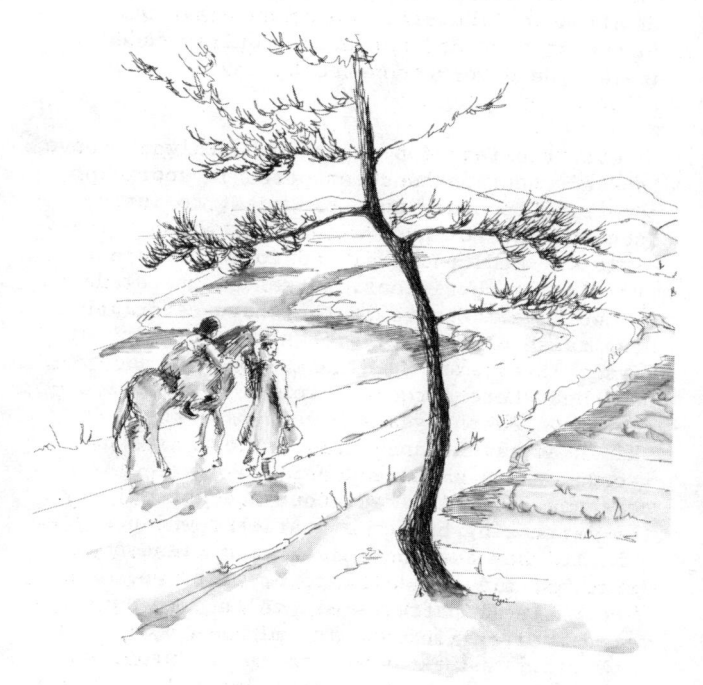

Kwangju Station was never the same, and the result was that Dr. R. M. Wilson established the first institution for victims of leprosy in all Korea in 1911. That same year Dr. Forsythe, weakened by sprue, retired once again. He never recovered and died in May, 1918.

Over the last 100 years such stalwarts have labored unnoticed and forgotten in scores of countries to stamp out epidemics, to introduce concepts of hygiene, to establish principles of medical care, and to launch the training of physicians, nurses and paramedical workers. Generally they have established hospitals--dispensaries or simple clinics at first, later small general hospitals, and here and there larger centers for medical education. As the years have passed their skills as clinicians and educators have been recognized as evidenced not only by the acceptance of medical science, and not only by the increasing burden of patients who have come to them seeking relief from illness and fear, but also by local governments who have adopted their patterns of health care and co-opted their trainees. The mission hospitals have grown and expanded and in the process something has too often been lost.

So today it is possible to speak of the transformation of lofty ideal into scientific institutionalism. The patterns of change were subtle and required several generations; yet one or more of the following processes were at work:

1. *The mission hospital became a teaching medical center.* It is quite normal that

medical missionaries should feel a responsibility to teach and to train. The Western physician has physical limitations; he cannot stay forever; periodic furloughs are needed and the work should not collapse in his absence. Further, how much greater the impact for health and for Christ if it could be multiplied by trainees who could implement the same skills and compassionate concern to a far wider segment of the population! Often the mission hospital was the first to become a medical school or the first to establish a training program for graduate physicians. But developing nations are prone not only to emulate such ventures but eventually regulate them. Sooner or later the numerous institutions which spring up either from that early mission hospital pattern, or from secular patterns learned by overseas trainees, must come under the jurisdiction of some government ministry or department. The pressures then begin to mount upon the Christian teaching center--of accreditations, of attracting qualified personnel, of complying with tax laws and complex and shifting legal requirements, or making ends meet in an increasingly competitive medical market. And many a hospital director or administrator, dancing on the spinning logs in the burgeoning stream of a health industry swirling through a strange culture, has slipped into the rapids or straddled the logs for safety.

2. *Compassionate outreach was diverted into clinical excellence.* Obviously, misinformed compassion has cost many lives. Christian medicine must be the best medicine possible or it will not be worthy of the name of Christ. Thus have many medical missionaries

reasoned, and for the most part quite properly, except that excellence is likely to become an idol. The pursuit of quality requires greater investment in plant, more elaborate facilities, and, particularly, more highly specialized medical personnel. Specialization is a part of Western medicine which has been implanted into developing countries around the world, and usually far earlier than actually needed by the health needs of those countries. It is a product of the international knowledge explosion in health science multiplied by the scholastic ambitions of the young brains in nations eager to catch up. And the mission hospital is often carried along in this tide, yielding to the current out of a fear that it might be bypassed in the thundering advance of science.

3. *Personalized care was changed to bioscientific impersonalism.* The dawn of bioscientific technology has placed a further stress upon patterns of health care within hospitals. Sterile technic and isolation rooms and visiting hours were antagonistic to the cultural patterns already. But now the superspecialists with their superdiagnostic gadgetry seek to impose their thought patterns upon the Christian hospital by fragmenting the patient and his problems, and introducing electronic refinements which are not only costly but tend to supplant the physician-patient relationship. The Christian hospital may possibly cope with these incursions, but may in the process lose its sensitivity to the persons it serves, and thus its opportunity for significant ministry.

4. *The witness of the heart is twisted into the arrogance of the mind.* How many great healing centers have lost their first love? How often does the founder's statue remain as the last tribute to the noble vision which sought to make Christ's love a reality in the experience of the suffering? Far too often the thrust of academic priority, the drive to professional excellence, and the pride of technologic progress have quenched the compassion that burned in the hearts of the pioneers. The generation of specialists in many a Christian center for healing is doubtless competent, yet no longer moved by the patient's cry.

These forces are not peculiar to the environment of Christian hospitals on mission fields. They are present in the historic flow of medicine around the world. The health industry in developing countries is promoting and exporting the technology of bioscience, but in so doing it is also exporting its consequences. Speaking at the 20th Congress of the International Hospital Federation, in Tokyo in 1977, Sir Gustav Nossal, Director of the Walter and Eliza Hall Institute of Medical Research in Melbourne, Australia, warned of the four dangers of the bioscientific revolution: increasing costs, depersonalization, overspecialization, and spectacularization.

The cost spiral is reaching such alarming proportions that at this writing the United States Government is seeking to regulate the purchase of expensive equipment by private hospitals. In 1935 the cost of health care per capita in the U.S. was $22.04; by 1973 it had reached $441.18,(7) and will soon reach 10% of the gross national product. This is the system which is being imposed upon developing countries. Nations struggling to stay alive are being sold linear accelerators, ultrasound equipment and computerized transaxial tomography (CT). One "CT" costs enough to build 10 to 15 Primary Care Centers which can cheaply control population growth, eradicate communicable diseases, and care for 90% of the health problems in rural areas of developing countries. As Health Planner H. B. Richter, from Brazil, asked at the Tokyo Congress, "Is there electronic equipment to fight hunger or illiteracy?"

Dr. Nossal's warnings about depersonalization, overspecialization and spectacularization emphasize the observations made earlier from the stance of a secular prophet. The electronization of medicine changes the healing art into a mechanical-mathematical exercise, and the patient's individual dignity becomes a casualty. Overspecialization works against a holistic (total) view of the patient. Spectacularization of crisis medicine results in disproportionate emphasis on "space-age" events such as organ transplants at the cost of investment in early diagnosis and preventive medicine.

"Better and better medicine for fewer and fewer people"--this is the indictment brought by many leaders in ecumenical agencies against the trends in Christian medicine around the world. The Christian Medical Commission of the World Council of Churches has much to say on this subject, but a few quotations from their 1973 Position Paper on Health Care and

The Dilemma

Justice will suffice to make their position clear.

> When the Christian Medical Commission was formed in 1968, its first major activity was to evaluate the existing patterns of relationship between church medical institutions and the people they served. . . Problems have now arisen which require new adjustments to changing conditions, without derogating in any way the contributions of the past.
>
> One sign of trouble has been our inability to keep up with the progressive effort to match in the overseas setting the qualitative improvements in hospital care which have characterized the scientific surge in world medicine. This has required a rapidly escalating investment in both facilities and personnel so that increasingly specialized physicians can work with more elaborate and expensive equipment. Hospitals are doing more and more for the same limited number of patients.
>
> The Commission's studies of the past five years have shown that the traditional hospital-based approaches have been both ineffective and inefficient.
>
> Our approach has been ineffecttive in meeting the total needs

of populations for both physcial and spiritual healing. Community surveys show that we reach only a fraction of the people in a hospital's orbit. It is no longer enough to say that our responsibility is only to provide a facility and then it is up to the people to come. . . Now that we have increasingly potent tools for both curative and preventive services, we must apply a whole new standard of priorities based on careful analysis of those approaches which are most effective in improving health.

The hospital-focused health care system is also inefficient. A clinical condition that requires massive investments--especially in the most precious commodity of personal time--could often have been prevented at a fraction of the cost. . . Our inefficiency is also evident in the way we use time within the hospital. Patients must invest inordinate amounts of wasted time in waiting while nothing is done. . . while the harassed doctor is trying to get through a phenomenal daily burden, most of which could be handled just as well by others. The fact is that elaborate hospital facilities are designed more to serve the professional convenience of overly busy physicians than the well-being of patients.

The Dilemma

> For Christians the most serious indictment of a primarily hospital-oriented health care system is that it is not only ineffective and inefficient but that it is also unjust. In fact, it is unjust partly because it is ineffective and inefficient. . . The definition of injustice here starts with the conviction that basic morality requires equitable distribution. The greater moral dilemma of medical care is to find the least unjust way to allocate scarce resources.(8)

So in one century Christian hospitals around the world have come to a point of crisis. Were their founders to walk through the terrazo hallways of the institutions they established what would they think? Would their initial amazement at the wonders of science give way to a gnawing sense of failure? Would they discern in the modern facilities that the patient is lost in the machinery? Would they find Christ's love still throbbing in the sterilized environment? Is the idea of the Christian hospital still viable or must the Church abdicate its role of healing? If the gospel proclamation is thus truncated how shall we be faithful to the Man whose love and power opened blind eyes and straightened twisted limbs and stanched hemorrhage? If the message of life abundant is thus diluted how shall we be true to the God-Man who said, "Greater works than these shall ye do, because I go unto the Father?"(9)

2

All we have willed or hoped or dreamed of
    good shall exist;
  Not its semblance, but itself; no beauty,
    nor good, nor power
Whose voice has gone forth, but each survives
    for the melodist
  When eternity affirms the conception of
    an hour.
The high that proved too high, the heroic for
    earth too hard,
  The passion that left the ground to lose
    itself in the sky,
Are music sent up to God by the lover and the
    bard;
  Enough that he heard it once: we shall
    hear it by and by.

                    Robert Browning,[1]
                    1812 - 1889

Why a Christian Hospital?

There are perhaps as many patterns of medical mission as there are medical missionaries. They vary from the jungle clinic to the gleaming hospital in terms of facilities; from the community-based preventive medical activity to the therapeutically-oriented teaching center in terms of program. As a veteran missionary remarked, "Both the strength and the weakness of missions is the individual missionary." The individual servant of Jesus Christ receives the call (which should be confirmed by some Church Board or sending agency acting on behalf of Christ's Church in order for the call to be scriptural). Thus set apart by his brethren under the guidance of the Holy Spirit he will go out to pioneer in new areas or to join the work of established programs or insitutions. But even when he becomes part of a team already on the field, it is often found that the medical missionary reserves the right to follow what he himself considers to be the Spirit's leading.

The thrust of this book deals with the idea of the Christian hospital. We will attack the concept, we will consider alternatives, we will seriously evaluate non-institutional Christian health programs, but we will start from the hospital idea not only because this is our legacy from the pioneers who preceded us, but also because this structure has had great impact for Christ in the past and because it is what we have before us to salvage or safeguard as a potential instrument for Christ in the future.

In doing this the author is acutely aware of the fact that Protestant Christian hospitals in the narrow sense may have ceased to exist in the United States. Church-related medical institutions still dot the map, and frequently carry a denominational label, but scarcely any of those of Protestant tradition are controlled by an ecclesiastical body. There are group clinics in which Christian physicians have bound themselves together in common purpose. But an important, nay, essential aspect of a Christian hospital is its *corporate* witness to Christ, and this implies more than the presence of a chaplain on the staff. The institution with which the author is affiliated requires all staff and employees to be professing Christians--a requirement which runs counter to the provisions of the Fair Employment Practices Act of the U.S. government. To what extent religious qualifications for entering into an association could be made practicable in the United States is not clear, but it probably relates to the distinction between public and private hospitals, and to the willingness of the institutions to forego Federal aid.

The basic question to which we will address ourselves in this chapter is "Why a Christian Hospital?". To say that a medical institution is or is not Christian is meaningless unless some criteria are agreed to, and this immediately implies selection of a purpose to be fulfilled. So "why" is more germane to our discussion than "what". We are here more concerned about the concept, the goal, even the ideal to be striven for than the degree of successs in achieving it.

In answering this fundamental question several unsatisfactory reasons have been set forth. The first of these is the "bait thesis." The mission hospital, some have said, is a sort of bait to allow fishers of men to hook patients into the Christian "boat". This most unfortunate concept stems from the legitimate concern for winning men to Christ. Perhaps basing their zeal upon Paul's assertion, "I have become all things to all men, that I might be all means save some,"(2) the advocates of the "bait thesis" would employ any or every means to bring men to the Savior, and medical care is considered no more than a means to that end. This viewpoint surely is dangerous. There is no objection to becoming fools for Christ's sake. There is no effort to escape the imperative of our missionary commission, nor the supremacy of the redemptive work of Christ over every other worthy activity in the Kingdom enterprise. The problem in this concept is not in the evangelistic zeal of those who advocate it but in the abusing of the objects of that zeal. It is a delicate line, perhaps, between sharing our testimony to Christ's redemptive power with those whom God has sent to us for loving

Why a Christian Hospital?

ministry, and utilizing our human ministry as a trap or a threat or a goad so that the afflicted might be captured during the crisis they face in the hospital. Nevertheless the proof of the method must be the sincerity of the commitment the patient is impelled to make. It is the love of Christ that should constrain men, and we dare not cheapen that love, even for evangelistic success.

A second concept is the "church hospital" idea: A Christian hospital is good medicine in an atmosphere of piety. The institution provides lay-support for the church and church-related vocations for its members. There is mutual benefit and mutual growth. In its most mature form this idea is expressed in the statement that "the hospital is the healing arm of the church." An organic relationship is established to formalize this concept, and the hospital regularly reports to the church conference or presbytery or assembly to which it is responsible. For its part the church supports the evangelistic program of the medical institution and through its representatives on the Board of Trustees seeks to safeguard the hospital's religious commitment. All these ideas are valid and workable. They simply fall short of what a Christian hospital is about.

The Christian hospital must be the Church at work, the Body of Christ in the world; and as such it cannot be contained by ecclesiastical structures nor defined solely on the basis of the close working relationship which should exist between the visible church and the hospital.

Closely related to the "church hospital" idea is the "monument thesis". In many developing countries, particularly where the Christian community is a small minority, great psychological support is given to those outnumbered believers by the presence of a hospital with a cross on it. It is the same reason for tall church steeples, perhaps. It gives us a sense of pride, of assurance, of being on the winning side particularly when the hospital which thus stands out in its community is doing a good job. But the monument idea is not only cheap but tricky, because there are always those who will attack it for its real or imagined failures, and the bigger the target the easier it is to defame.

In the preceding chapter we quoted several paragraphs from the 1973 Position Paper on Health Care and Justice of the Christian Medical Commission, quotations in which the entire hospital-oriented health care system is indicted as being inefficient and unjust. Dr. Michael Wilson, a former medical missionary to Ghana and now Lecturer in Pastoral Studies, might be considered a spokesman for this "Geneva Viewpoint" (the headquarters of the World Council of Churches and the Christian Medical Commission is in Geneva, Switzerland). Dr. Wilson suggests that our health care system is a victim of a built-in contradiction--that you obtain health by the eradication of disease. "A system of medicine founded upon knowledge of disease does not produce health: it can only discover more disease and create the very needs which it is supposed to meet."(3) He cites three assumptions which are powerfully conveyed to all who take part in the life of a hospital:

a. That the cure of disease is more important than the care of people;
b. That the provision of health is the task of experts;
c. That death is the worst thing that can happen to a person.

He makes a noble appeal for redefining the role of the hospital as follows: The primary task of the hospital is to enable patients, their families, and staff to learn from the experience of illness and death how to build a healthy society."(4)

In the next chapter I will attempt to answer more fully the Geneva indictment of inefficiency and injustice, drawing upon the history of the hospital where I have served since 1954, Presbyterian Medical Center, in Jeonju, Korea. In this chapter we are dealing with the more basic task of considering the reason for the existence of the Christian hospital itself. Dr. Wilson's thesis is that the role of hospitals is secondary to the health of society and that they should function as supportive agencies in the context of that priority. In criticizing the three "powerfully held" assumptions of the "Hospital Establishment" he has scored a telling blow which needs to be struck against entrenched attitudes. But these assumptions should not be prevalent in Christian hospitals unless they have drifted far from their founding purposes.

I find more difficulty with the assertion that the eradication of disease is ineffective in producing health. If I've got a cancer I want it removed or destroyed. If I've got an abscess I want the pus drained. If my heart is failing I want those drugs which can reverse the process. Dr. Wilson's reasoning only makes fragmentary sense in terms of community health and (to some extent) in the prevention of disease. He is saying that the individual's crisis is relatively unimportant; his illness is the result of his ignorance of health. It is to the well we must carry our efforts, creating a system of medicine founded upon knowledge of health in order to eliminate the need for curative efforts. This is my understanding of the Wilson thinking.

It must be admitted that hospitals too often failed to meet the needs of the community in their orbits, that "intolerable health conditions" are sometimes perpetuated around Christian medical institutions, that the health of the society has too often been beyond the scope of their felt responsibility. But Dr. Wilson's thesis contains two fundamental flaws, one medical, and one theological. First, it seems to assume that all disease is preventable by health education. This is far from the case. Secondly, it sacrifices the worth of the individual to the welfare of society. Christian hospitals can be faulted for not going out into the community to find the afflicted who might never come in; they cannot be faulted for upholding the value of human life.

What is a healthy society? In an underdeveloped society the immediate threats are epidemic disease and malnutrition. As we move up the development scale chronic illnesses such as tuberculosis, parasitic infestations, and "poor men's cancers" become major

Why a Christian Hospital?

problems. Later, cardiovascular disease and the "rich man's cancers" assume importance. But there is no such thing as a healthy society in this world, only degreees of health, for we live in an abnormal universe, a universe tarnished by the Fall, and therefore bound to the processes of physical death. In the strictly physical sense the job of physicians is to postpone death. But the Christian physician has much more to give: he is a disciple of the only one who can truly heal, the Physician of the Soul.

It is shallow to propose that we can establish a system of medicine which ignores disease in its effort to create health. It is specious to state that discovering disease is fruitless, that it simply creates need. The creation of those forces within society which enhance nutrition, hygiene, and healthful life-styles are surely the hospital's business. But to place the long-range objective of a healthy society in top priority over the life and death crisis of the hour, over the destiny of the individual who comes pleading for life and for relief from suffering, to turn aside from the anguish of one human being for reason of a commitment to the community's welfare is not an option available to a sincere disciple of Jesus Christ.

Why the Christian hospital? It is not primarily an evangelistic stratagem, though it should be among the most effective methods of witnessing the love of God in Christ. It is not an instituion to enhance the prestige or growth of the Church, though it should generally be instrumental in church growth.

It is not primarily designed to teach the community how to build a healthier society, although it has a tremendous responsibility here. The Christian hospital derives its reason for existence from one historical fact alone: Jesus healed. I follows that the gospel of Jesus cannot be complete without that compassionate ministry. Look for a moment at our Lord's medical value system, if you will. Walking through the countryside, through towns and cities he encounters men suffering disease--some acute, some chronic, some congenital, some acquired, some major, some minor. He stops. He may make it an occasion to forgive or to exhort, but he never passes by. He heals all who come to him for help. To the leper asking to be cleansed: "I will; be clean."(5) To the man with the withered arm: "Stretch forth your hand."(6) To the paralytic: "Take up your bed and walk."(7) To the man in the tomb: "Lazarus, come forth."(8)

Why the Christian hospital? Because Jesus Christ healed, and in so doing demonstrated that our God is compassionate, that He is moved by human suffering. And therefore Christ's disciples must seek to be instruments of healing, in one or more of the various avenues available for medical ministry. And one obvious pattern is the hostel for the sick which allows medical disciples to concentrate their time and facilities to do the most for the seriously ill. We now recognize that it is but one part of a pyramid of health care; but it remains essential. It is to be an exhibit, a demonstratrion, of the character of God.

Why a Christian Hospital?

Peter wrote that God's "divine power has granted to us all things that pertain to life and godliness, through the knowledge of him who has called us to his own glory and excellence, by which he has granted us his precious and very great promises that through these (we) may. . . become partakers of the divine nature."(9) The theological implications of this statement are tremendous, but I would only emphasize the central idea that God supplies all we need to allow us to become partakers in his very nature, participating in his character, sharing in his being. A Christian hospital can become this.

In fragmentary ways, for moments in its corporate existence, the medical institution which bears Jesus' name may become His temple, demonstrating the desire of God to dwell among His people to rescue and restore. It is never an accomplishment, yet always the goal; never the completed reality, yet often a true experience: the disinfected wards become a sanctuary; the bedside, a Bethesda; surgery becomes Solomon's porch. It is at once an ideal to be pursued and a command to obey; that in claiming the Name we should reflect Christ's compassion and exhibit God's mercy in order that men by faith might live.

3

The Father and his Troubadour sat down
Upon the outer rim of space. "And here,
My Singer," said Earthmaker, "is the crown
Of all my endless skies--the green, brown sphere
Of all my hopes." He reached and took the round
New planet down, and held it to his ear.

"They're crying, Troubadour," he said. "They cry
So hopelessly." He gave the little ball
Unto his Son, who also held it by
His ear. "Year after weary year they all
Keep crying. They seem born to weep then die.
Our new man taught them crying in the Fall.

"It is a peaceless globe. Some are sincere
In desperate desire to see her freed
Of her absurdity. But war is here.
Men die in conflict, bathed in blood and greed."
And both of them beheld the planet bleed.

                            Calvin Miller[1]

A Philosophy of Medical Mission

Until the Second World War the medical policy of the Southern Presbyterian Mission in Korea was to maintain small hospitals in each of its major stations: in Chonju (as it was then spelled), in Kunsan, in Kwangju, in Soonchun, and in Mokpo. This effort was dependent upon medical missionaries to man each of these posts, and one consequence was that some hospitals were often left unmanned during a missionary's furlough or when illness forced him to return to America. Dr. G. T. Brown commented on this problem in his history of the Korea Mission:

> An acute problem in the medical work through the years has been the rapid turnover among the medical personnel. Because of overwork and the frustration of being required to do so much with so little, the loss of doctors has been proportionately greater than that of evangelists. Up to the present, only one Presbyterian U.S. missionary doctor has been able to serve in Korea until retirement age.(2)

A Philosophy of Medical Mission

So through long years was the medical work continued at these outposts despite the perennial uncertainty of maintaining a medical staff, interruptions caused by illness and destruction by fire. In Chonju five different doctors served intermittently until Dr. Lloyd K. Bogg's directorship of 16 years, which ended when all missionaries withdrew at the brink of the Pacific War. In Chonju the record is as follows:

1897   Dr. Mattie Ingold began a women's dispensary in a thatched roof house purchased for $24.

1902   A new building erected for Dr. Ingold by Mr. Harrison.

1904   Dr. Wiley Forsythe became director of this unit, but was injured by bandits in 1905 and his work was cut short.

1911   A 30-bed hospital was built and was directed by Dr. Thomas Henry Daniel, who resigned in 1915 for health reasons. From this time forward it came to be known as Jesus Hospital.

1915   Dr. M. O. Robertson became director of the Chonju Hospital, resigned in 1918.

1922   Dr. H. L. Timmons served as director of the hospital, resigned in 1926.

1924   Dr. Lloyd K. Boggs was appointed to the work in Chonju and served until the hospital was closed in 1940.

1934   Hospital burned to the ground, was rebuilt as a 40-bed unit the following year by Dr. Boggs.

In 1947 Dr. Paul S. Crane returned to Korea as the first new medical missionary to arrive on the field after World War II. At the Mission's request he and Miss Margaret Pritchard, R.N., toured the Mission to reevaluate opportunities for medical work and recommended that "instead of returning to the pre-war plan of a general hospital in each station, the mission consolidate its medical program with a major effort "concentrated in one well-equipped properly staffed medical center at Jeonju, where adequate training of interns, nurses, and technicians would be accomplished."(3)

My wife and I joined the team at Jeonju in April 1954. A new wing was under construction which would shortly increase our bed capacity to 150. The Nursing School had reopened after the Communist invasion. The number of refugees was an index of the social chaos which followed the Korean War, and our hospital was a daily battlefield against unimaginable disease and neglect. In this situation we attempted to create a training hospital, providing post-graduate medical education to physicians in medicine and surgery, while establishing a laboratory training course and continuing the nursing school. I contracted tuberculosis and Dr. Frank Keller, a pediatrician, came to help.

A Philosophy of Medical Mission

In 1960, Korean Specialty Academies were organized in every major specialty, and each of us became accredited by national examination in order to authenticate the training of interns and residents. Although Presbyterian Medical Center had chronologically pioneered the post-graduate training concept, when the idea was adopted nationwide it was with such zeal that specialization became the name of the game, and no provision was made for training general practitioners.

Meanwhile two other medical programs were underway. In Kwangju the Graham Memorial Hospital, which had served primarily as a center for tuberculosis patients under Dr. Herbert Codington, broadened its scope to become a general hospital while continuing its tuberculosis program after Dr. Ronald Dietrick joined the staff in 1962. Near Soonchun the Wilson Leprosy Hospital also assumed a new role as a rehabilitation center after Dr. Stanley Topple assumed leadership there in 1960.

By 1961 it was evident that the building erected in Jeonju by Dr. Boggs 26 years previously, while sturdy, could never serve as the basis for a modern teaching center. It was a jack-leg conglomeration of leaking pipes, blocked drains and electrical improvisation. There was no room for expansion. Foreseeing the dilemma Margaret Pritchard and I requested that this hospital be designated the beneficiary of the 1965 Women of the Church's Birthday Offering. Paul Crane returned from furlough in 1962 and for three years the missionary team gave intensive study to the need for expansion. The Mission consented to transferring to Presbyterian Medical Center the site of an old primary school which was to be closed. In 1964 we applied to the Evangelical Central Agency, in Bonn, Germany, for a major matching grant.

As we look back on those years of dreaming, planning, fund-raising, negotiating and praying we feel a certainty that God was at work in removing obstacles which were humanly insurmountable, in order to bring about "The Miracle of Dragon Head Ridge"--the new medical center which stands at the southern perimeter of Jeonju today. But during those years of waiting we could not clearly foresee the outcome. Later we realized that the delay was a necessary part of God's plan. For one thing, it allowed the multiplication of the funds donated by our home church. Interest rates were abnormally high during those years. Paul Crane and our Administrator, Merrill Grubbs, decided to bring our entire building capital to Korea for investment in Korean banks, and the result was that eventually the Birthday Offering funds were more than doubled, and actually exceeded the matching grant of 5 million Deutschmarks when this was finally approved late in 1969.

But perhaps of even greater importance, during those years of waiting, Dr. John Wilson came to serve with us and launched us in a new direction, into the field of community health. By the time we had been assured that the new medical center could be built we had made a corporate commitment to alter the nature of our basic program, not by curtailing our teaching activities, but by accepting as of equal importance our role in providing

A Philosophy of Medical Mission

health care for the rural communities which surround us.

When Paul Crane resigned in 1969 after 22 years of service, the German grant was yet in doubt. During the summer months that followed his sudden departure the Lord removed the obstacles to the grant's approval, and on October 10 we received the joyful news. Space will not permit me to elaborate on the numerous events which filled the strenuous years of planning, construction, and reorganization between 1969 and the present, yet I must pay tribute to many fellow-workers who poured out their lives and energy for the fulfillment of our common dream: to establish in Southwestern Korea, a healing center worthy of the name of Jesus which it bears. Here we would erect a center no less compassionate than professionally competent; no less evangelical than scientific. Here we would bring together a witnessing community of medical disciples of Christ who by their concern for the individual in trouble, as a person, and a member of a family and of a community, would exhibit the character of God himself.

To summarize, what then are the characteristics we would pursue in order to be worthy of the Name:

1. *We should be people-oriented rather than disease-oriented*. Dr. Micheal Wilson's warning is appropriate. With medical success comes the demand for more service for more people. Shortly after moving from the old hospital we found that we were treating three times as many out-patients, and twice as many in-patients as in the old hospital. The work

load itself poses a threat to our purpose. It is for this reason that daily chapel services, weekly Bible study groups, and religious emphasis weeks are part of our tradition. We are aware that we require God's strength in the face of such heavy demand. Our strict religious requirements for employment are part of this same concept. No one is qualified to serve who does not himself recognize Christ as Saviour and Lord.

2. *God's truth and mercy should govern our corporate life.* We make no distinction between the validity of the truth God reveals through His Word and the truth He discloses through scientific inquiry. Because He is Creator and Sovereign we accept the risks of trust, principle, and openness in a society of suspicion, relativism and intrigue, confident that these risks are known to Him who has power over human events. Because God is Redeemer and the Forgiver of Sins we must be merciful toward patients and forgiving to one another. What we teach and what we practice must correlate.

3. *We must be faithful to the gospel of Jesus Christ.* We have been entrusted with the work of reconciliation. Evangelism is everybody's business. The lives entrusted to our care have eternal dimension. We dare not lose sight of a patient's ultimate need for the saving grace of Christ. As we broaden our responsibility to the communities about us we must yet uphold the value of the individual, inviting his participation in deliberations which affect the health of his village and his family.

A Philosophy of Medical Mission

4. *We would become the healing arm of the Church*. Although this concept is not a definition of our purpose it is important. The hospital completes what may be lacking in the church's ministry in making the message of abundant life in Christ germane to the existential predicament of men in trouble. The relationship of the Church to Christian institutions of healing must be organic and supportive. It must not become sectarian or dominating. The Church has a stake in the effectiveness of our witness; we have a stake in the growth of the Church.

5. *The community is our medical parish*. Not only the patients who come to our doors seeking help; not only those who come as to a court of last resort; not only the emergencies and those with advanced or complex medical problems; not only the desperate who come to us shall comprise our responsibility. There are those whose ignorance and poverty are the barriers to receiving health care; who resign themselves to needless suffering because there is no man to feel outrage for their chronic despair. These also are our parish. We must go to them, to treat their afflictions and to prevent the diseases to which their survival life-style has made them prone, teaching them to be responsible, to plan and to hope.

This is the framework for our work and witness. Our consciences require us to be competent clinicians concerned with the whole man. At the same time our consciences demand our participation in providing primary health care for the community. We are stretched between our concern for the individual and our

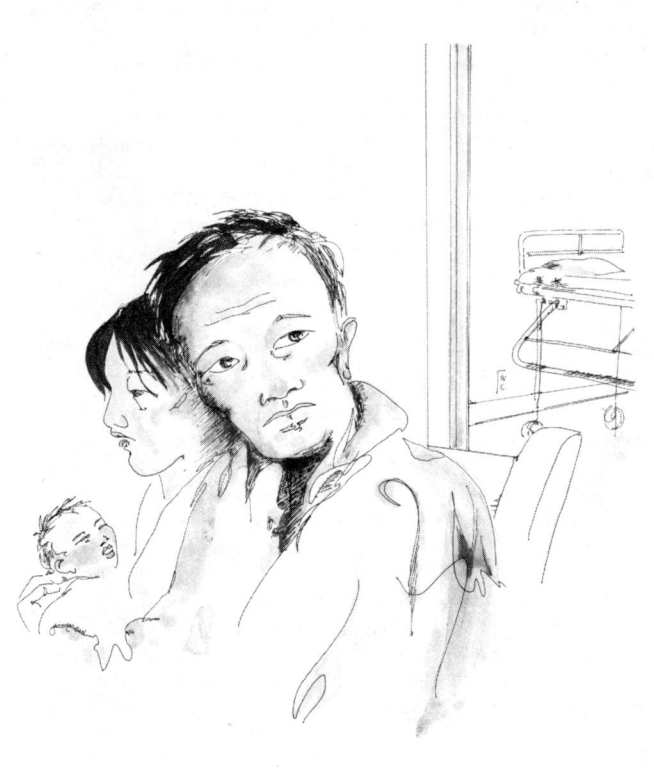

concern for the community in which he lives. We must recognize that this tension we feel is our normal stance.

Yet we wrestle with daily problems in seeking to implement these five concepts of people-oriented medicine practiced by a Christ-witnessing community which exhibits God's truth and mercy as the healing arm of the church, not only to the individual but to his community as a whole. Here are some examples of the practical problems we face in this implementation: a) How do we individualize the financial evaluation of a patient who is unable to pay for his care? b) How much time can we devote to teaching when the clinic waiting areas are full? c) How do we exercise judgment in the purchase of life-saving equipment which increases our costs and hospital charges and thus may limit our ministry to the poor? d) How much effort should be devoted to cure and how much to the prevention of disease?

We do not pretend to have all the answers; we are often baffled, perhaps to fight better. The Christian Medical Commission charges that the hospital pattern is inefficient and unjust. Let us evaluate our own record on the basis of these criticisms.

First as to the charge of *injustice*, we would make the following observations:

*We never turn away an emergency. What sort of a Christian witness is it to refuse to save a life on the pretext that the cost of saving that life might prevent 100 from becoming sick? Shall we withhold life-saving help in a real crisis because the cost might help prevent a theoretical crisis? I know of no Christian clinician who could live with his conscience so bound. We must, we can only assume that God places our skills at the scene of human need for the purpose of alleviating that need.

*There is no such thing as free medical care. There are free patients, but no free medical care. Someone, somewhere must pay the cost. At our hosptial the bulk of the cost of free work is borne by the paying patients. This Robin Hood principle not only works but can be employed with some measure of reliability to assure a substantial number of poor patients of needed medical care.

*Community Health work costs. We have emphasized this as an integral part of our work. The paying patients support this program also. We have been studying other community health ventures in Korea. None of them is self-supporting, and all programs which are not hospital-based depend upon grants from abroad.

Secondly as to the charge of *ineffectiveness*. It is true that we meet total needs of only a fraction of the people in our hospital's orbit, and that serious disparity exists as to the proportion of urban vs. rural population which avails itself of medical care. We would make the following observations:

*Although the proportion of rural patients which make up our clientele has decreased from 52% to 44% between 1956 and 1975, the rural population has decreased from 75% to 66% in the same period. The proportional

A Philosophy of Medical Mission

changes are almost identical. The critical factor is our capability for individually processing and compassionately meeting the needs of the farming population which comes to us. An effective Social Service Department is crucial.

*Should every general hospital adopt a population area over which it would extend primary health coverage a substantial improvement in the health care delivery system could be effected. In time we hope to expand the size of the population group to which we offer primary health care, but this is contingent upon the sense of responsibility which the specific communities shall accept for their own welfare.

*When and at what level will government responsibility supplement or supplant the role of voluntary agencies? We believe we can work with many government plans to alleviate the lot of the most destitute segments of society, not only in our present community health areas but throughout the province.

As emphasized in the Statement of Health Care of the Presbyterian Church, U.S., "to heal means far more than to cure."(4) Our primary task is to heal, and this requires the work of Christ, the physician, in the life of my patient. We have been entrusted with the message of reconciliation and healing, but the patient's destiny depends upon an act of faith in the Great Physician who stands behind me.

It becomes apparent that healing may take place when cure is not possible. A polio

victim's withered leg may be stabilized with
a brace, but substantial disability remains.
Plastic surgery may do wonders but cannot restore
the beauty of youth. A cancer patient's
disease is often impossible to eradicate. It
is deceptive to state that God empowers people
to be whole or that God desires health
for every man, unless we go beyond the physical
context. Healing and health cannot be
set forth as goals merely in the physical and
psychological orders of life. When we remember
that Jesus is a life-giving spirit and
that His resurrecting power transcends the
physical definition of health we come closer
to the meaning of wholeness--God's perspective.

More than once I have heard it said that,
"Health is not a privilege but a right."
While sympathizing with this noble sentiment
I must say that the Scriptures offer little
support to this viewpoint. Rather we read
that the entire creation is in bondage to decay
so that "all created life groans in a
sort of universal travail."(5) It is specious
and shallow to think that all physical
illness is against the will of God, or that
physical health (or the lack of it) is a
measurement of spiritual health (or lack of
it) even for Christians. I believe our compassionate
Father agonizes over the suffering
of all of His creatures, but His eternal
righteousness and love are not always manifested
as physical healing in this life.
Suffering is part of life: "For this slight
momentary affliction is preparing us for an
eternal weight of glory beyond all comparison."(6)
So it is preferable to state that
health *care* should be every man's right, and

that those of us who do enjoy health are under obligation to participate in the sufferings of those who do not have that privilege, so that as Christ's suffering abounds His comfort may also abound. Physical pain and every form of human suffering are distressing to God, but there is no evil as great as rebellion against Him.

Dr. Michael Wilson is certainly right in his observation that death (physical death) is not the worst thing that can happen to a man. The worst thing is spiritual death, eternal separation from the glory of God. Every effort we make to minister to the afflicted must be in the framework of that truth.

4

Christianity cannot ultimately be judged by a mere comparison with other creeds. Its tenets are so absolute that it can only in the last resort be judged as true or false. The statement that in Jesus God was revealing himself to man; that in the death of Jesus God was reconciling man to himself; that in the resurrection of Jesus God was declaring the conquest of death forever; such claims cannot be reckoned as better or worse than another creed. They can only be judged as true or false.

                              T. M. Kitwood[1]

The Truth Beyond Faith and Science

A visitor from our General Assembly Office of Evaluation in America sat in my office during a discussion with our hospital leadership. Each of our division chiefs had sought to express how he or she envisioned the distinctive character of Jesus Hospital: a place where Christians of every denomination and physicians from every medical college could join together in comon purpose to serve their Lord; a place which had helped establish the dignity of nursing; a place of unprecedented evangelistic opportunity to the nearly 100,000 persons who come for care each year; a place where science and faith meet without conflict to express God's truth. The visitor, a woman elder and clinical psychologist, remarked, "There is no model in the United States for what you're trying to do here." Perhaps not. But undoubtedly around the world many Christian medical institutions at various stages of development are grappling with these same issues. Even in America conscientious Christians in medicine are surely seeking ways to create agencies which express corporately God's redemptive love. This small book

The Truth Beyond Faith and Science

is for all those concerned with medical witness in every continent. Our experience and perspectives may not apply in many situations. As representatives of a program in a rapidly developing country we can identify both with the disadvantaged and with the advanced. In this context we set forth our convictions concerning the Christian hospital as an exhibit of the character of God.

There are at least four dimensions to this concept:

1. It should be a testimony to the truth beyond faith and science;

2. It should be a repository for the concept of human worth;

3. It should be a witness to the preeminence of Christ;

4. It should be a demonstration of a lifestyle of love.

In this chapter we will think about the first of these criteria. We are talking about truth not as some romantic ideal but as something that exists. Undoubtedly it is possible to be involved in planning the life and work of a Christian hospital without articulating a Christian world-view, without thinking through the relationships between doctrine and disease, without considering the interaction (or confrontation) of faith and science, without pondering what link may exist between the created universe and the predicament of one afflicted human being. Undoubtedly it is possible to be medical

scientists or health workers with a sheen of
religion or a pattern of piety which fulfills
the formal requirements for participation in
Christian medicine. But an institution whose
leadership has not achieved a Christian world-
view is vulnerable. It has clay feet and
will soon compromise its spiritual purpose,
for it cannot withstand the onslaughts of
either scientism or secular existentialism.

   The history of Western Man, according to
Schaeffer, is a philosphical journey during
which two of the three classical principles
of philosophy were abandoned. These three
principles were: 1) *rationalism*, the idea
that man, beginning absolutely and totally
from himself, can gather information about
particulars and from these formualte universals; 2) *rational logic* as the process whereby
man carries out this quest; and 3) *the construction of a unified field of knowledge* as
the goal of this pursuit. It is beyond our
purposes here to discuss the history of philosophy except in relationship to the question
of the existence of ultimate truth.

   Yet every thinking man has a world-view,
and as Christians we must recognize ourselves
as philosophers in the fundamental sense of
loving wisdom or searching for truth. The
three principles set forth above characterized western philosophy at the outset of the
dialogue between its Greek roots and the
Judeo-Christian view.

   Let us bear in mind that all of the ancient philosophers of the West "acted on the
basis that man's aspiration for the validity
of reason was well founded."(2) Logical

thinking presupposes the methodology of antithesis, wherein we define things by contrasting them with their opposites: "If a certain thing was true, the opposite was not true. . . That is the way God made us and there is no other way to think. . . The basis of classical logic is that A is not non-A."(3) The basic problem to which the philosophers addressed themselves was posed by Boethius (480-524): "What is the relation of universals to the individual material things that exemplify them, and to the human mind that knows them?"(4)

Augustine (354-430 AD) is said to have established the bridge between Greek and Christian thought. He introduced the concept of *derived existence* as the link between universals and particulars, that is to say, that the existence of the created derives from God's being. In contrast, Aquinas (1225-1274 AD) maintained that active intellect is not God derived or even a direct manifestation of God, but is on its own, "and has all it takes to fulfill of itself and by itself the purpose for which it was created."(5) Thus Aquinas launched the idea that the human intellect is autonomous. This gave impetus to rationalism and divorced human inquiry from any reliance whatever upon sources of information other than those acceptable to man's intellect. Aquinas did not himself question the existence of revealed truth, but the "enlightenment" which grew out of his thinking eventually did. Gradually the realm of nature (the particulars in Greek thought) expanded to devour the realm of grace (the universals of Hellenistic philosophy) so that man was left with nothing which gave cohesion or meaning to his knowledge. Schaeffer proposes that until Kant's day Western man held on to the hope of finding an answer that would encompass all of life. With Hegel, antithetical thinking (Principle Two) was put aside and Western man was left with no rational basis for knowing. With Kierkegaard and existentialism he gave up the pursuit of a unified field of knowledge altogether (Principle Three). The quest for ultimate truth has been abandoned and man is left without absolutes. Schaeffer maintains that "this change in the concept of the way we come to knowledge and truth is the most crucial problem. . . facing Christianity today."(6)

The significance of these developments for a Christian hospital is profound. Few institutions place science and faith in so close a juxtaposition. Secular hospitals may remain silent on moral issues or may acquiesce to the social consensus, as has occurred with "abortion-on-demand." On the other hand the institutional church may or may not speak out, but does not itself become involved in the ethical (and legal) crucible, except through the consciences of its medical membership. In a Christian hospital belief in absolutes is no theoretical exercise. It affects the lives of children unborn, the therapeutic struggle in the intensive care unit, and the consciences of young doctors and nurses who are formulating their own professional creeds.

In order for a hospital or any other human agency to exhibit the character of God there must be some understanding about God's nature, about His work in the cosmos, His attitudes toward His creatures, His intervention on their behalf, and about His empowering men to become God-like (loving, altruistic, upright, merciful). It should be understood that God is not part of nature or of a closed system within the universe, but stands outside it as its Author and Creator. Four steps may be discerned whereby we may exhibit God's truth.

First, there must be a commitment to the existence of absolute truth. This may seem redundant, but liberal theology with its Tillichian emphasis upon God as unknowable, "wholly other," and the impersonal "Ground of Being" would cast grave doubt upon man's being able to apprehend any ultimate truth with certainty. The historical Christian perspective is that absolute truth stands squarely upon the character of God. This God both creates and communicates, and thereby what is factual derives both from the evidence of creation and from the information He reveals to man about the cosmos, about history, about man and about Himself. God is ultimately the source of all that is true. As Professor Arthur F. Holmes has put it,

> If we confess that God is the all-wise Creator of all, then he has perfect knowledge of everything men ever sought to know or do. The truth about the physical order is known perfectly to Him, the truth about man and society, and the truth about everything we ever wondered about in our most perplexed moments. The early church fathers summed this up in what has become a guidepost for Christian scholars ever since--*all*

> *truth is God's truth, wherever it
> be found."*(7)

The second step is the cultivation of the integration of faith and science. Revealed truth and scientific truth are both expressions of God's creativity and communication. Pascal observed that one cannot search for or discover truth without in some way learning something about its Author. He was deeply impressed by "the mathematical orthodoxy of the physical world."(8) One of the early modern scientists, Kepler, stated that science is "thinking God's thoughts after him."(9) And Schaeffer has grasped a fundamental fact of history in stating that modern science was possible only because of the Western concept in which the subject (the investigator) and the object (the experimental data) were understood to have the intrinsic correlation which comes of both being parts of the created universe. "The whole area of science turns upon the fact that (God) has made a world in which things are made to stand together, that there are relationships between things."(10)

The Christian scientist or physician has not necessarily resolved every problem in Scripture any more than he would claim to comprehend all the scientific facts of the universe. He simply believes that in God all the facts will ultimately cohere. Neither the biblical revelation nor scientific inquiry provide an exhaustive source of all truth. God communicates truly but not exhaustively. To know anything exhaustively we must be infinite, as God is infinite. Just because truth is not exhaustive does not mean it is not true truth. Holmes summarizes the matter succinctly: "If all truth is God's truth and truth is one, then God does not contradict himself, and in the final analysis there will be no conflict between the truth taught in Scripture and truth available from other sources."(11)

The third step in the process is the elaboration of a Christian medical world-view based upon God's truth. It is beyond our scope to present a working philosophy for every situation, but certain concepts are central and will dictate our medical priorities. These deal with the cosmos, with man, and with the existence of evil.

a) *Cosmos.* The Christian believes in a personal universe. "This is my Father's World." The vast complexity of the created order testified to his Father's unfathomable intellect. The extravagant swaths of color on the Western sky at sunset, the trembling flower in the breeze, the song of the nightingale testify to his Father's love of beauty. The mathematical interplay of physical forces and the vast sweep of the galaxies speak to him of God's order and infinity. For some nature is cruel and impersonal, and no one may be exempt from its fury. But the Christian knows that nothing can separate him from the love of God in Christ, no landslide, no earthquake, no tidal wave can change that eternal relationship.

The Christian knows also that he is God's deputy on earth, not by accident but by appointment: made the steward of the planet, all its plant and animal life, all its resources, all its energy, all its people. He is to subdue the earth, have dominion over nature, and be the keeper of his brother. The hospital is a microcosm of that stewardship. Here he dares to employ macroshock for defibrillation, radioisotopes for scanning a hidden organ, the dog lab for testing vascular technics, gamma rays to destroy cancer cells.

The cosmos is not only God's creation and man's trusteeship but also the laboratory for his intellect and curiosity. Every leaf, every fossil, every chromosome, every star commands his attention and stimulates his mind: why, how, when, where? The scientist of Judeo-Christian tradition stands before God challenged--to discover the causes of disease and the means to health through the exercise of the intellectual powers God gave him and this challenge is the stuff of life because there are answers, because God made the universe with a system that can be understood even by finite minds, because it is not just a product of chance and because there is order and not chaos in nature. So in the hospital earnest men can tax their brains in making an obscure diagnosis or proposing an elaborate program of therapy basing their reasoning upon the predictability of normal or abnormal physiology, the reliability of anatomic relationships, and the restorative healing process in the human body--why? Because God fashioned the living organism and its intricate biochemical functions, because God is at work sustaining the universe and healing the patients' wounds.

b) *Man*. "What is man that thou are mindful of him or the son of man that thou dost care for him? Thou has made him little less than God, and dost crown him with glory and honor. Thou hast given him dominion over the work of thy hands. . ."(12) The Bible tells us that man is a creature of peculiar majesty, the image-bearer of God, fashioned for a glorious destiny. The Bible tells us also that man is a tragic failure, a rebel against his Creator, who though he may reach the planets of this solar system cannot govern himself. The Bible also tells us that man is the object of God's providence and grace, "providence that limits evil and preserves man's personality," and "grace that restores God's image and sanctifies human powers for God's glory."(13)

In a later chapter we shall deal with the mystery of human worth, but it is man's potential that we must consider here. I am reminded of Hammarskjold's phrase, "To love life and men as God loves them--for the sake of their infinite possibilities."(14) Man was created for a glorious destiny, for immortality and for eternal joy in God's presence. Every man has that potential of fulfillment or its anithesis in his hands. No man is programmed. Every man is free to choose and is responsible for his choice. This potential for glory begins even before birth. Jeremiah was consecrated to the Lord's service while yet in his mother's womb. David testified that his fetal parts were recorded in God's book before his birth. The abortion lobby may succeed in the Supreme Court but physicians who seek a consistently Scriptural world-view cannot dismiss these references to the potential and the sacredness of unborn human life.

I remember an infant born with a ruptured omphalocele at our hospital. The parents refused to allow surgery. I checked with our lawyer to see whether we could take such a case to court and was informed that the hospital by Korean law could do nothing. The child died of peritonitis in three days. Such incidents are not rare for infants are virtually non-persons until given a name in the social psychology of this country. Often a child is not named until the 100th day of celebration, and during this period the infant is in limbo, proving its ability to survive, perhaps, proving its right to personhood. In our early days in Korea it was customary in the society for only one of twin infants to be breast-fed; the healthier looking child was given the breast and the other one only water until it died. Only by insisting on the chance to artificially nourish the second twin in the hospital—at no expense to the family—could we salvage its life. And how many abandoned babies did we nurse to health and eventual adoption! We have learned never to tell the family that a child has a 50% chance at survival through such-and-such an operation or therapeutic effort because the Korean mind-set is to look at such figures in the reverse: 50% chance of death. Much better to take the child to die at home.

The point of all this is that the Christian physician must take his stand against whatever the concensus or the culture may prescribe when human life is at stake.

But it is not simply a matter of struggling against those forces which cheapen human life.

The Truth Beyond Faith and Science

There is a more subtle yet more prevalent problem: the problem of meaning for life, meaning which often is most keenly sought when life hangs in the balance. Here I recall my own failures most clearly. I have been with patients shortly before their death, and I confess that as a doctor it is profoundly difficult to minister to the patient's spiritual needs. First, there is the urgent effort to save the life, often against insurmountable odds. At this moment it seems in the worst taste to speak to the patient about Christ lest we convey to him the desperateness of his situation. So his consciousness gradually fades, and the family--if nearby--begins to wail, and the brief moment of truth passes forever. And depressed by failure or remorse we busy ourselves with the next crisis: our duty is to the living.

So by philosophical pretext or psychological mechanism we continue to fight on against the powers of darkness, seldom availing ourselves of the power of prayer, seldom having the courage to place the patient's immortal destiny in its proper priority above everything else we would do. Yet there have been times when the light in dying eyes shined with hope, when I could pray with a patient before the house staff, times when the truth beyond faith and science became the principle and the policy of eternity's moment.

c) *Evil*. How few physicians have resolved the problem of evil in the world! I know of experienced cancer specialists who succumb to profound depression after twenty or thirty years of struggle. I myself may become deeply discouraged after a day in Tumor Clinic. As

C. S. Lewis wrote, "Cancer and cancer and cancer. My mother, my father, my wife. I wonder who is next in the queue!"(15)

What has helped me the most in this regard is Francis Schaeffer's analysis of the Eleventh Chapter of John. Jesus arrives at the home of Mary and Martha and seeing Mary weeping "was deeply moved in spirit and troubled." He wept. Later coming to the tomb he was "deeply moved again." The Greek word used in these two passages is not found elsewhere in the New Testament. The word is *embrimaomai*, which means "to snort in spirit"--a furious inner anger. And as Guinness has commented, Jesus, entering his Father's world as the Son of God, "found not order, beauty, harmony and fulfillment, but fractured disorder, raw ugliness, complete disarray --everywhere the abortion of God's plan. The death of Lazarus symbolized the accumulation of evil, pain, sorrow, suffering, injustice, cruelty, and despair. Thus, while he was moved to tears for his friends in sorrow, he was also deeply moved by the outrageous abnormality of death." (16)

Now, I can understand this outrage, because I have felt it in confronting cancer. In "Does My Father Know I'm Hurt?" I described it as the personification of evil, a prototype of Satan, and I have alluded to the need for the therapist to maintain the tension of indignation against his evil antagonist as he mounts a life and death struggle upon his adversary.(17) But Schaeffer goes beyond describing the outrage of Jesus, the outrage of God, to make clear what a relief it must be to us to know that God does feel outrage against the evil in the world--that what is, is not *right*; and therefore when we struggle against the evil in the world we are not struggling against God's will but rather joining Him in the divine conflict.(18)

For many the first ten chapters of Genesis are semi-mythological. But the practical consequences of setting aside this ancient part of the Scriptures is not only to discard the doctrines of creation, of man being God's image-bearer, and of his trusteeship over the earth; but also to create a formidable theological and philosophical problem. Without the Doctrine of the Fall there is no answer to evil in this world, no basis for understanding that God's perfect creation was forever tarnished, that our universe is abnormal, that sin and death have entered the world through man's rebellion. I prefer to accept the biblical record on faith not only because I hold a high view of scriptural authority but because it correlates with my life's experiences as participant in the cosmic struggle for men's minds. I believe there is a supernatural sphere of spiritual conflict between the forces of Satan and the hosts of the Lord. As Paul phrased it:

> We are not engaged in a human conflict; we are not involved in a worldly war. The weapons of our warfare are not of the flesh, but divinely powerful for the destruction of fortresses. We are destroying speculations, we demolish every proud obstacle to the knowledge of God, to bring every thought captive to Jesus Christ.(19)

The Christian hospital is a battleground in this war. Illness, pain, despair, the temptation to disregard human life, the shame of poverty and the fear of death, the pressures of overwork and the stress of anguished choice: here is the arena where those forces are engaged. Everyone of us becomes consciously a participant in the conflict, and if we do not have clear convictions about God's truth, about His available power, about His resources of love and mercy and justice and faithfulness we are struggling with our hands tied behind our backs, which is like trying to perform surgery with one hand.

Finally, there must be a reordering of medical priorities. God's truth is radically divergent from the thought patterns of society. Every human being bears the stamp of God's image. All of creation is placed under human trusteeship. The entire universe is ours to explore. Man was created for glory and is the object of God's redeeming grace. Every human life is sacred in His sight. Health is not the ultimate standard but rather proximity to God. We live in an abnormal cosmic order where evil often prevails. God feels outrage and so must we. The ultimate struggle is spiritual. The cross of Christ is the central fact of history. Jesus Christ is the measure of all things. He would not leave my patient desolate.

Every professional pattern may be overturned. Away with the specialist's fragment; we are dealing with total persons precious in God's sight. Away with bioscience; we are talking about health and life. Away with the spectacular; we are talking about the real.

5

Our western way of life has come to a parting of the ways; time's take-over bid for eternity has reached a point at which irrevocable decisions have to be taken. Either we go on with the process of shaping our own destiny without reference to any higher being than man, deciding ourselves how many children should be born, when and what varieties, which lives are worth continuing and which should be put out, from whom spare parts--kidneys, hearts, genitals, brain boxes even--shall be taken and to whom allotted.

Or we can draw back, seeking to understand and fall in with our Creator's purpose for us rather than to pursue our own; in true humility praying, as the founder of our religion and civilization taught us, Thy will be done...

We can survive energy crises, inflation, wars, revolutions and insurrections, as they have been survived in the past; but if we transgress against the very basis of our mortal existence, becoming our own gods and our own universe, then we shall surely and deservedly perish from the earth.

Malcolm Muggeridge[1]

A Repository for the Value of the Individual

One of our missionary friends tells the story of a train wreck which occurred many years ago outside the town of Hillsboro, North Carolina. The town's people gathered around the scene of the accident and were told by the authorities that a man was still trapped in the wreckage. The town doctor and the sheriff, at some risk, went into the twisted pile to see if the man could be extricated from the weight of the box cars which were crushing him. It was impossible to free him; and after some time, the effort was abandoned. The sheriff addressed the crowd of townspeople: "It's all right. It's just a hobo." And from the midst of the wreckage came the gasping cry of the injured man: "I ain't a hobo. I'm Jesse Smith." And then he died.

For nearly 25 years I have lived in a culture which traditionally has not accepted the principle of intrinsic human worth. This is not to say that Asians do not have the same human aspirations, the same natural desires for love and security, the same inclination to pursue happiness.

The Value of the Individual

In America we have learned that when a man has no self-respect, he cannot respect anyone else. When he devalues himself, he devalues everyone. Christ said, "Love your neighbor as yourself."(2) This implies that both your neighbor and you, yourself, are worth loving.

In the Orient, the matter of self-respect is dealt with by the creation of a vertical system of prestige and of an elaborate pattern of amenities. Every person spends a great deal of time learning where he fits into the totem pole or how he can rise to a higher peg. But this does not create appreciation for every man's worth--quite the opposite. Why, for example, should a physician, a graduate of six years' premedical and medical education, get up out of bed at two o'clock in the morning to treat a beggar who fell into a fire during an epileptic convulsion? The individual has never had intrinsic value in the East because there has never been a basis for such a concept. Yet the basis for human worth in the West is also being eroded away. Today the individual in the West is crushed by depersonalizing forces which are greater than those he has ever experienced. It has produced a climate of despair which pervades much of society. Let us examine some of the forces which undermine the worth of human life. The first of these, the population crisis, is a world-wide phenomenon, more acute in the underdeveloped areas of the world. The second and third apply principally to Western culture, but have counterparts in two additional factors which are native to the East.

1. *Population Explosion*: According to a *Reader's Digest* pictograph, it took four million years for the population to reach 800 million by 1776.(3) In the 200 years since that date it had grown to 4.1 billion, and at the current rate of growth (doubling time of 38 years) it will reach 8.2 billion by the year 2014. Each 24 hours the world population increases by 295,602 persons at this rate, which works out to almost 7 persons every two seconds. In Korea a valiant effort has been made to slow this rate of growth reducing the annual increase from 217% to 1.9% per year. Even at this rate the doubling time is only 38 years.

I was born in Florida, and the fondest recollections of my youth are days of running on deserted Gulf beaches, the powdery white sand crunching under my toes, the whole expanse of sky and waves and shore for the moment mine--no other footprint, no other body under the sun. Some years ago, I spent two years in New York City during my training at Memorial Hospital. Once or twice on a summer afternoon we ventured out to the Long Island beaches. The jumble of human bodies cluttering the sand was such that we could scarcely reach the water. And I fear that sooner or later all of America's beaches will be despoiled by the clutter of our soaring population. In Asia, on the other hand, it is not a question of beaches. In many areas, it is impossible to get out of sight of other people. South Korea is the third most densely populated nation in the world; and by a strange coincidence, in the Korean language a word for "privacy" does not exist. In the glut of human life, whether in America or in

The Value of the Individual 63

Asia, the individual man feels no longer unique; he has become *nameless* in the mass; and this sense of being superfluous has inevitably altered the core of his thinking. Unconsciously, he comes to regard life as cheap.

2. *The Technologic Age*: The second force crushing the individual in America and Western Europe is the age of technology. Man, in choosing efficiency, security, and success as his ultimate criteria for achievement, first created the machine to do his work, then to communicate for him, then to think for him. Human inquiry led to scientific discovery which led to an explosion of knowledge which led to the need for data processing which led to centralized computerized control of many of the mechanisms of society. *In* the process man becomes victim *of* the process, and loses his sense of meaning for life. One by one his technical skills are replaced by more efficient electronic circuits. More and more his performance is evaluated on the basis of impersonal criteria, is tabulated by number, and is fed into data storage facilities. Day by day his thinking is patterned by mass communication media which establish the norm for society.

The result is *programmed man*. He may be able to maintain some freedom of choice, but his initiative is blunted; and his sense of controlling his destiny is lost. There are those who openly advocate technocracy. It seems but a small step away. Technocracy is government by technicians, in which all economic resources and hence the entire social system are controlled by scientists and engineers. In the military-industrial complex, the age of technocracy may already have arrived. Gradually, man, his creative skills suppressed by automation, the content of his conversation patterned by television, the options of his destiny controlled by computer, ceases to find interest in life. If the population explosion has robbed him of his sense of uniqueness, the technological age has robbed him of his sense of purpose. He is not only nameless but also meaningless in the world.

3. *The Deterministic World-View*: The third force which crushes the individual in the latter 20th century is the deterministic world-view which largely pervades Western society. The philosophy of Rousseau, Freud, and Dewey proclaims that man is only the product of his heredity and environment. This view is inescapable if man begins with himself, rejecting every other source of ultimate truth than that which he can learn from his own experience. Having learned that nature is governed by laws, if he then assumes that there is no other source of truth he will gradually place every aspect of life and knowledge under the control of nature, surrendering ultimately his body, mind, and spirit, even his personhood, to mathematical laws of chance and physiochemical laws of cause and effect. Man then becomes a machine, and because this knowledge is intolerable he is in despair. There are, in this world view, no moral attributes. Love no longer exists. Beauty is simply an arbitrary neurophysiological perception. To his namelessness and meaningless must be added the most damning result of all: man is become lifeless.

The Value of the Individual

4. *The Supremacy of Nature*: Among the major differences which affect the thought patterns of cultures is the contrast between the Western and Eastern attitudes toward nature. As mentioned in an earlier chapter, the biblical injunction to subdue the earth and have dominion over it has helped the West not only to explore the planet to discover its laws and its secrets but also to employ these in subjugating nature's forces to human control. The East traditionally has never spoken in such terms, but rather of harmonizing oneself with nature's forces, to establish a pattern of mutual coexistence, as it were. Yet nature is generally acknowledged to have the upper hand. Centuries of disasters of floods, earthquakes, and famines have taught the Oriental to acquiesce to natural forces. Further, the absence of a personal God in Eastern thought has led to the attribution of divine will not only to "heaven" but to an innumerable pantheon of other natural deities--yet these are always contained within the natural order. No fundamental distinction is made between man and other forms of natural phenomena. And here as in the technocratic consequence described above, the options are few. Human purpose in the East is often limited to the question of survival and to maintaining some kind of continuity, with one's ancestors and through one's offspring. The family becomes supremely important, but there is no value attributable to the life of someone outside the clan, someone to whom no obligation is owed or from whom any favor can be expected.

5. *Religious passivity*: It is no accident that the Eastern religions have become

attractive to the "lost generation" in the West. When man is reduced to a machine, when absolute truth is unknowable, when all of life is the product of mathematical chance, when man is reduced to a zero he has attained essentially the state of Buddhist philosophy would have him attain: nirvana, the bliss of nothingness. There is neither good or evil, cruelty or non-cruelty, joy or sadness, only the peace of withdrawal from the world with its pain.

Namelessness, meaninglessness, and lifelessness. Whether the meaningless came from technologic or from philosophic depersonalization the result is the same. Whether the lifelessness came from deterministic or from religious reductionism the result is the same.

My own work is among cancer patients in rural Korea. It may seem an unlikely place to fight a battle for human worth. In this country, a cancer diagnosis is an automatic death sentence and the survival economy makes no effort to salvage human life beseiged by such a hazard. The cancer victim is relegated to being an unperson, along with the abandoned infant, the beggar, the convict, the prostitute, and the "leper." And the whole thrust of our purpose in establishing a Christian teaching hospital in the Orient will be found in opposing, in protesting, in decrying this silent inhumanity of man toward man. For this reason the cancer struggle, for this reason the midnight surgery, for this reason the repeated mouth-to-mouth respiration to oxygenate an infant with tetanus whose life hanges by a thread for days on end.

The Value of the Individual

The value of the individual has no basis in world economy, no basis in technologic progress, no basis in either modern or ancient philosophy. In the Scriptures of the Old and New Testament only is there hope of human dignity:

> When I look at the heaven, the work
> of thy fingers,
> the moon and the stars which thou
> has established;
> What is man, that thou are mindful
> of him,
> and the son of man that thou
> dost care for him? (4)

> Are not five sparrows sold for two
> pennies?
> And not one of them is forgotten
> before God.
> Why, even the hairs of your head are
> all numbered.
> Fear not; you are of more value
> than many sparrows. (5)

The Christian hospital is surely not the only defender of the dignity of man. But because it is inextricably involved in human life processes it assumes major importance to the preservation of the Christian value-system. In this sense it may be called a repository of human worth. There are three concepts in God's Word which undergird this doctrine of individual worth. Each is a teaching with regard to the nature of God, for human value is always derivative. Wherever the Christian gospel is preached these three ideas should be included. Wherever the Bible is seriously studied these ideas will spring forth.

1. A PERSONAL GOD

Francis Schaeffer writes, "As a Christian I know who I am, and I know the personal God who is there."(6) He exists not merely as a transcendent First Cause but as a Person. We must understand that the existence of human personality is dependent upon the personhood of God. Scriptures tell us that when God breathed into man's nostrils the breath of life he became a living soul. To argue the creationist view or the theistic evolutionist view is unimportant provided we agree that man as a person began at the point in time when God provided that "mouth-to-mouth" insufflation from His own life. This is the key to human identity.

Every patient is God's image-bearer (how easy to say, how difficult to remember in the crowded clinic). Every man, woman or child waiting to be called, every resigned or anguished or anxious face that comes before me bears the impress of God's life-giving spirit. Will I receive them and treat them thus? Christ went further. He took the position of the patient's surrogate. "What you do to him you do to Me. If you treat him ill it is Me you insult. If you treat him mechanically it is Me you disdain. If you love him you love Me." Can I possibly remember that each face in the long parade is Christ, my patient?

God's personal nature not only bears upon my attitudes to the patient but upon my relationship with God Himself. If the essence of my life is a template of the Father's character, there should be a normal urge to companionship. As foreigners walking down a street

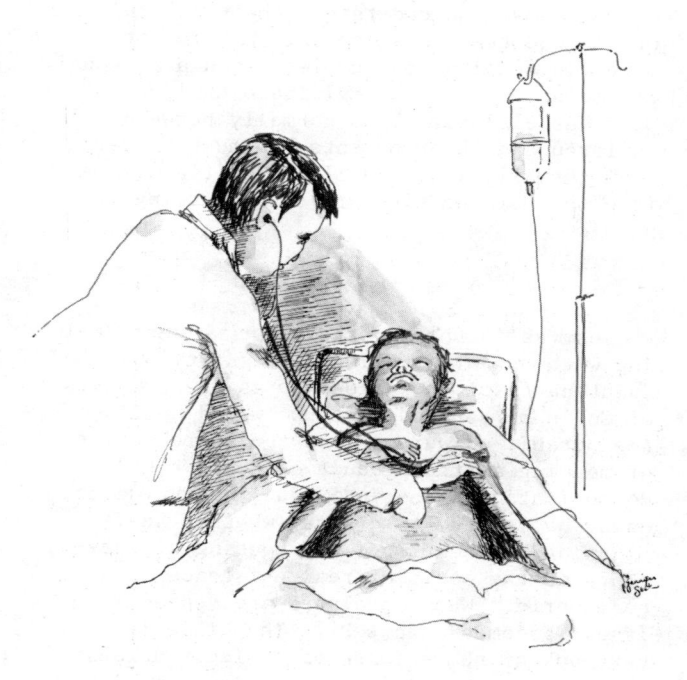

in a crowded city we can hardly resist the
urge to greet an American face. "Where are
you from? How long have you been here?" We
have common roots, we are hewn from the same
rock. How much more should this urge exist
between those who understand their supernatural
origin and their Originator. We are not
merely disciples, but copies, with a personal
resemblance: we are legitimate children of
God. As dialogue flows normally between
children and their parents, so must prayer
flow normally in our daily activities as we
face the perplexities or joy of working with
people.

2. A KNOWABLE GOD

Just as in the first concept we were dealing with the affirmation of identity and the
maintenance of companionship as the products
of God's personhood, here we would consider
the pursuit of purpose and the apprehension
of meaning as the product of God's truth and
communication. The individual has value because he is free to choose (whether he is
planning his next move or choosing his destiny) on the basis of real existence in a
real world. When absolutes are denied life
itself becomes a fantasy. The Bible is a
textbook of the science of choice. Abraham
chose to answer God's call, sojourning 1,000
miles across Mesopotamia and Canaan, and the
result was that a nation was founded. Jacob,
Joseph, Moses made choices which had perpetual consequences. Joshua led the people of
Israel to stand on two mountains in northern
Palestine to reemphasize their freedom to
choose between the blessings and the curse of
God. And throughout the Scriptures we

encounter the recurring theme: "Choose you this day whom you will serve."(7) Man is not programmed, and no one knows this better than the physician of integrity who has the courage to reevaluate his choices and learn from them: which choices saved life, which choices failed. If critical choices could be tagged with radioisotopes and detected by a probe, few places on earth would show a higher scintillation count than an active hospital.

Among the "Ten Commandments for House Staff" which I use in my orientation message for interns, two are relevant to this concept:

"All my life was spent in preparation for this day;"

"Today is the patients's golden day."

The Christian physician may not shrug his shoulders with a "Que sera, sera." Every decision counts. We are purposeful beings living in a real world, because God Himself is purposeful, because God works and acts in history and made us of the same stripe.

3. A REDEEMING GOD

Man has value and dignity not only because he is fashioned in God's image, not only because he is the object to whom God has communicated truth, and a being able to make significant and purposeful decisions in a real universe. He also has worth because when the great experiment failed and man rejected the contract with his Maker, God refused to cast him out, but instead took upon Himself the consequences of man's rebellion through the cross of Christ.

Strangely enough most folk cannot figure out why they feel restless and alienated from themselves. Whether in the East or West, they will pursue a solution to this central dilemma of existence through the long corridors of life but never come to grips with the cause. In the West this pursuit is attributed to guilt-psychology; in the East to fear-psychology (since absolute moral categories have traditionally not been recognized). Today the East-West distinctions are becoming blurred, yet whatever the terminology the vacuum is still present in the human psyche, the God-shaped vacuum which only God can fill, the vacuum which is created by sin, by falling short of the divine plan.

And then comes illness, striking in the small hours of the night or insidiously wearing away the body until the point of desperation is reached, and the patient comes pleading for life in the last stages of peritonitis, or septicemia, or cancer. "Give me to live!" they cry in Korean. The issue at the moment is not whether hospitals are ineffective for maximal health care delivery. The problem of the hour is not whether the center of gravity for health should be the community or the institution. The crisis is intensely personal: one lost soul crying out in the dark. By whatever other criteria Christian hospitals are inefficient or expensive or inappropriate, they are made to respond to this call. Most of the staff is in bed, the night duty technicians and supervisor and house staff and attending physicians make up the small skeleton crew grappling with this one life, yet this is the hospital's golden hour, and that crew's range of motion coincides with the arc of destiny for one human being. Can they be trained to recognize that it is not only a countdown for life but for eternity? For if Christianity is true, that soul, because it lives forever, is of more value than the hospital itself, more than the state, or the nation, or even a civilization, for as C.S. Lewis has observed, that individual "is everlasting and the life of a state or civilization, compared with his, is only a moment." (8)

6

I see His blood upon the rose
    And in the stars the glory of his eyes.
His body gleams amid eternal snows,
    His tears fall from the skies.

I see His face in every flower;
    The thunder and the singing of the birds
Are but His voice--and carven by His power
    Rocks are His written words.

All pathways by His feet are worn,
    His strong heart stirs the ever-beating
        sea.
His crown of thorns is twined with every
        thorn,
    His cross is every tree.

                      Joseph Mary Plunkett[1]

Witness to the Preeminence of Christ

When we discussed the principle of God's sovereignty over all truth in the Fourth Chapter we omitted from our presentation a corollary principle for which we are also in debt to Professor Holmes, the principle of the *unity of truth*. This principle is derived from the "cosmic Christ" passage in the first chapter of Paul's letter fo the Colossians:

> He is the image of the invisible God, the first-born of all creation; for in him all things were created, in heaven and on earth, visible and invisible, whether thrones or dominions or principalities or authorities--all things were created through him and for him. He is before all things, and in him all things hold together. He is the head of the body, the church; he is the beginning, the first born from the dead, that in everything he might be preeminent.(2)

The Preeminence of Christ

"In Him all things hold together." A physicist can better describe how much energy is released when a nucleon is released from an atomic nucleus by fission. The nuclear particles of atomic substances are held together by extraordinary attracting forces, which can be overcome by nuclear bombardment releasing energy in accordance with Einstein's classic formula, $E = mc^2$. But here the scriptures make a superlative claim regarding the entire structure of matter as it exists in this universe. It is held together by the dynamic cohesive force of Christ. This claim goes so far beyond our usual picture of the God-Man; so far beyond the customary dimensions of our thinking that it "blows the mind." Christ is not only the unifying cosmic force but the unifying cosmic truth. In Him "are hid all the treasures of wisdom and knowledge."(3) All of our knowledge of anything comes into focus around this fact. As Holmes put it, "The truth is a coherent whole by virtue of the common focus that ties it all into one." (4)

This cosmic Christ is not only preeminent in creation, the cohesive factor in the galactic reaches of space; he is also preeminent in redemption. This rank is accorded him by the Godhead: "in him was all the fullness of God pleased to dwell." And the focus of the preeminence is Christ's work for mankind. The cosmic forces are at his command but he would reconcile men to God "making peace by the blood of his cross."(5)

As the primeval creative force Christ established the universe and even now upholds it by his dynamic will interacting in the

physical forces of nature. For this reason
we look to him as the unifying principle in
science and in morals, the final absolute
which undergirds truth. In the practical
sphere of life he becomes our basis for policy. As the superlative redemptive power
Christ is the incarnation of God's wisdom and
mercy which conceived of the cross as the ultimate means of salvation, having power to
reconcile all things, whether in heaven or
earth. In the practical sphere of witness
this cross must be central to our message.
Let us then apply these two aspects of Christ's
preeminence to hospital life, first in terms
of institutional policy, and then in terms of
our evangelistic thrust.

I. *PREEMINENT IN POLICY*

Hudson Taylor, the great missionary pioneer
of China from the last century, set forth a
premise regarding God's Kingdom enterprise
which bears serious consideration: "The Lord's
work in the Lord's way shall never fail to
have the Lord's provision."(6) During my
tenure as director at Presbyterian Medical
Center I have consciously tried to make this
a guide to practical policy. One of our employees had a scroll printed with these words
in Korean, which hangs in my office. I have
failed on many occasions, but next door to me
is the office of my colleague and brother in
Christ, Merrill Grubbs, Hospital Administrator, who will gently chide me when he feels I
have not been consistent with that principle.
What is the Lord's way of working?

God's Word tells us that He does not work
through human energy, not through the energy

of His own disciples except insofar as by
faith they reckon themselves dead unto sin
but alive unto God through Christ. According
to Schaeffer, there is only one "how" in God's
methodology. "It is the power of the crucified, risen and glorified Christ, through the
agency of the Holy Spirit, by faith."(7) In
True Spirituality, Schaeffer sets forth Luke
9:22-24 as the scriptural basis for God's
methodology. Here Jesus initially speaks of
His own work, then of that of His disciples.
First, "the Son of Man must be *rejected,
slain, raised,*" in that order. Then, speaking
of his disciples' work, Jesus said they must
each one *deny himself, take up his cross,
follow Christ,* in that order. Renunciation,
crucifixion, new life in Christ. Saying "no"
to the secular systems of society, saying
"yes" to Christ at whatever price is required,
and thus becoming alive to God. If God is to
empower men to do His work He will do it in
His way. Without a cross there can be no
resurrection. Without the death of the old
man there cannot be new life in Christ. Without renunciation of all other gods Jesus cannot become Lord in our hearts. Unless we are
crucified with Christ we cannot be raised
with Him. But once raised with Him we are to
reckon ourselves dead to sin and alive to God:
God can work. Christ can reign. The Spirit
can empower.

These tough Anglo-Saxon words that strike
out at us from passages such as Luke 9 and
Romans 5 and 6 leave us little "room to wig-
gle." The concepts are so simple yet so profound, so easy to grasp, so difficult to put
into practice in the daily decisions of a human organization in the modern culture of the

latter 20th Century. Is it possible? I will suggest some of the areas in which we have attempted to put the idea to work, confessing in advance that there are borderline situations ("gray areas") where it has been difficult to be sure we were doing the right thing, and have proceeded on faith and prayer.

In the construction of the hospital itself there were many opportunities for compromising principle. The greatest of these occurred when the government failed to keep its promise regarding the duty-free importation of $600,000 worth of construction supplies, and demanded an equal amount in duty charges. At this point the construction was well along: four of the six floors had been shelled in.

It was tempting to respond to the invitation to bribery. We refused to do this, and God provided for us a man of influence who expended that influence to gain fair consideration of our request. He was a Christian assemblyman in the National Legislature. His father had been a mission chauffeur many years before, and had died at Jesus Hospital of tuberculosis before the Second World War. And his eldest son, Mr. Yongjin Kim, had never forgotten the kindnesses of the missionaries and staff toward his father 30 years previously. This national legislator protested our cause. Day after day he visited the Ministry of Health and Social Affairs, demanding that the government abide by its promise. From the Minister of that bureau to the clerks at the lowest echelon he demanded explanations. For almost two weeks he caused upheaval until the decision had been made to grant duty-free import of the hospital construction supplies. It was an unprecedented event.

Mr. Kim lost the next election, and shortly after was killed in an automobile accident. For a brief time he came on the scene to serve as God's answer to our dilemma. His ultimate commitment to Christ led him to risk his political career to save the future of our hospital. And yet this answer to our problem had been in preparation a generation before. Thus through events that none of us knew about God had prepared a provision for a need on condition that we take our stand against the system (renunciation), except whatever the consequences might be (crucifixion), and cast ourselves upon God.

The work of this 269-bed medical center is multifaceted, encompassing clinical care, post-graduate and nursing education, maintenance engineering, comprehensive evangelism, cost accounting, community health. In every area of our corporate life we are endeavoring to make Christ central, to consider the cross our normal method of operation. In financial policy this means choosing compassion before solvency. In personnel policy this means giving priority to Christian commitment over intellectual excellence. In medical policy it means placing the whole patient above the narrow scope of a specialist's expertise. In community health policy it requries listening to the community representatives rather than arbitrarily imposing upon them the health program we think they need. The cross as a policy in institutional management—the phrase may sound strange, beyond reason in terms of management theory. But if PMC is to live up to its Korean anem, "Jesus Hospital," it cannot function with the priority system of the world. It cannot plan to survive on human energy. As Schaeffer has commented, "The Lord's work done in human energy is not the Lord's work any longer. It is something, but it is not the Lord's work."(8)

II. *PREEMINENT IN OUR MESSAGE*

In the previous chapter the Christian premise that individual life has value was established upon the character of a God who is personal, knowable and redeeming. Because He is personal man has personality, a personality that can be creative like the Creator's, and loving like his loving Father. Because God is knowable, that is to say, because he reveals truth about Himself, man can know true truth, and this makes all of his choices meaningful. His life can be purposeful as God's life is purposeful. Because God is redeeming, because He loves His creatures to the extent of an agonizing substitutionary death at Calvary, man has an answer to his fundamental dilemma of guilt and fear, and can be saved. He can be restored into fellowship with God by recognizing the sin which caused God to suffer, and by accepting in faith Christ's work on the cross as "the sufficient and necessary sacrifice for his sins." These concepts are all embodied in Christ's words: "I am the way, the truth, and the life; no one comes to the Father but by me."(9) Because Christ is the life, we regain our lost identity ("I am the good shepherd; I know my own and my own know me.").(10) Because Christ is the truth we find purpose and meaning in God's communication to us ("If you continue in my word. . . you will know the truth and the truth will make you free").(11) Because Christ is the way we have salvation from sin and access to

The Preeminence of Christ

God ("We have confidence to enter the sanctuary by the blood of Jesus, by the new and living way which he opened for us through. . . his flesh.").(12)

The problem in hospital evangelism in a non-Christian culture is the matter of making the message simple yet germane to the patient's understanding of his own predicament. No one method is applicable to every person nor appropriate at every occasion. Establishment of a personal relationship between the witness and the patient is essential.

A grateful patient went to the hospital office and asked the staff there what sort of gift his doctor would like to receive. The office worker replied, "The greatest gift you can give him is to become a Christian." "Is that so?" the patient exclaimed. "I'll take my whole family." And he did, all of them becoming active in the church.

A young woman with a sarcoma of the leg consented to have her leg amputated after praying with the surgical staff. She was already a Christian. After the operation she witnesses to the patients on either side of her in the six-bed ward. "I don't care if I've lost my leg so long as I've got Jesus." Two women in that ward accepted Christ through that testimony.

A farmer with gum cancer was given a New Testament by his doctor while he was getting elective post-operative radiation therapy after undergoing a "Commando" procedure (a radical surgical operation on his mouth and neck). A month later he returned for his Tumor Clinic appointment. "Did you read your Bible?" he was asked. The patient stood up and, with a smile and the characteristic tongue-tied pronunciation produced by his surgery, recited John 3:16.

I prefer to emphasize witnessing as a somewhat broader concept than evangelism, one that must include evangelism, but which also includes the entire scope of our concern for the patient. It begins when he registers in the clinic, it should be evident by the kindness with which he is treated in the x-ray department, in the laboratory, in the office. It should continue throughout the doctor-patient relationship, and particularly through the nurses' bedside contact. Smiles, reassurance, prayer, concern, individual interest: these are the essential ingredients to hospital preevangelism. But the message itself in propositional form must not be neglected.

"*You are valuable* in God's eyes. You were created to have fellowship with Him and to live with Him forever. He is holy. *You have a problem.* If you do not know Christ you have missed God's purpose for you, you have made yourself your own god, you have shown God ingratitude. You are responsible before Him. Perhaps this pain and suffering are for a purpose--to help you recognize your problem: you are not fit to live with God. *There is a cure* for your soul-sickness. Jesus Christ, God's Son, took upon Himself the consequences of your sin and gives you His righteousness. He can change your curse into a blessing. But you must put your trust in Him."

The Preeminence of Christ

Gentleness, concern, sincerity—these are essential. Every member of the hospital staff should ideally be able to witness. The chaplain's help or that of his assistants should always be available. But every disciple of Christ on the employee roster should know the mystery of "holding this treasure in earthen vessels, to show that the transcendent power belongs to God."(13) Finally, the witness must be validated by love, love toward the patient and love among the brotherhood of faith. But that is the subject of the next chapter.

"I am the way, the truth and the life." Jesus Christ is the focus of our evangelism just as he is the focus of our policy and the center of our corporate life: in all things Christ preeminent. "For in him all the fullness of God was pleased to dwell, and through him to reconcile all things. . . by the blood of his cross."

7

She called from her cell,
"Let me give you a rose,"
To the cold tract-man
In his Sabbath clothes.

And the tract-man said
To the one gone mad,
"How can you give
What you never had?"

"As you give Christ,"
The madwoman said,
"While love in your heart
Lies cold and dead."

Harry Lee[1]
1874-1942

The Corporate Life-Style of Love

Administration of an institution with 575 employees is no picnic. There are times when major differences occur between the management and the regular employees. In the Spring of 1977 such discord did occur, and it severely tested much of what we have worked for--the concept of the witnessing community, our unity in Christ, and our corporate love toward one another. Restraint, patience and love won the day through the work of the Holy Spirit, and we have all learned something from the experience. Walking down from the hillside where dawn Easter services were held I found myself alongside the employee who had been the instigator of the unrest. He said, "I have caused you much anguish lately." I replied, "The important thing is that in the love of Christ we can solve these problems."

In an organization such as ours the love of Christ cannot be a sentimental platitude or a theoretical idea. It's what holds us together. But it takes openness, fairness, communication, common worship, and common concern to make this love real.

The Corporate Life-Style of Love

A family of nearly 600 representing two cultures, four nationalities, seven major denominations and innumerable schools and colleges can be expected to have occasional upheavals, given the traditional proneness to factionalism in Korea. Certain cultural factors militate against oneness: strong ties of loyalty to school and region; the absence of privacy and confidentiality; and the unusual sensitivity to inequities or disparities, real or imagined. Under the circumstances we believe the best policy is openness. Intrigue is the name of the game in society but we will be open, all books ready to audit, all records available for perusal. Fairness and justice are difficult principles to implement because they ultimately depend upon someone's value system. As a safeguard all decisions regarding personnel policy (the "point system", regulations, promotions, etc.) are made by the Executive Committee by democratic vote. Communications up and down the table of organization are extremely important. The labor unrest mentioned earlier in this chapter occurred primarily because communications had not been adequately maintained. But the most important factor in upholding our family relationship is our common worship. Daily chapel for all employees consumes many man-hours but it is this which draws us together, which focuses our minds upon Christ, and which empowers our service through the inner working of the Holy Spirit. It also draws us closer to the Church, whose ministers regularly serve as devotional speakers.

Employee policies must be conciliatory and sensitive to personnel needs. Through a credit union sponsored by the hospital many of our folk have recourse in the event of sudden financial need. The credit union manages the sundries shop and the tea room, arranges annual picnics and athletic events, and operates a beach cabin for vacations.

Over 70 ladies representing all protestant denominations in Jeonju donate their time to the Volunteer Service Society. Some of these women, whom we refer to as "Pink Ladies" because of the color of their uniforms, have given over 1,000 hours of time running a book cart, serving tea or water to patients in the clinic, writing letters for bed-ridden folk whose disability or disease handicaps them, folding gauze, feeding, running a nursery for visitors, and performing numerous other jobs which no one else can find time for. As I have told them, they fill in the love-vacuums which we leave behind us in our busy-ness.

The nurses run a bazaar each year to raise scholarship funds for employees under stress to educate their children. A biweekly newspaper carries news of hospital and personal events. At times of personal grief, Christian Koreans have a remarkable way of supporting and comforting each other.

Another source of inspiration is the hospital choir. Koreans have beautiful voices, and love to sing. The hospital choir blesses us at many special occasions, competes in nationwide contests, and produced a record for our 80th Anniversary. I have often been moved to tears by the loveliness of their praise and devotion.

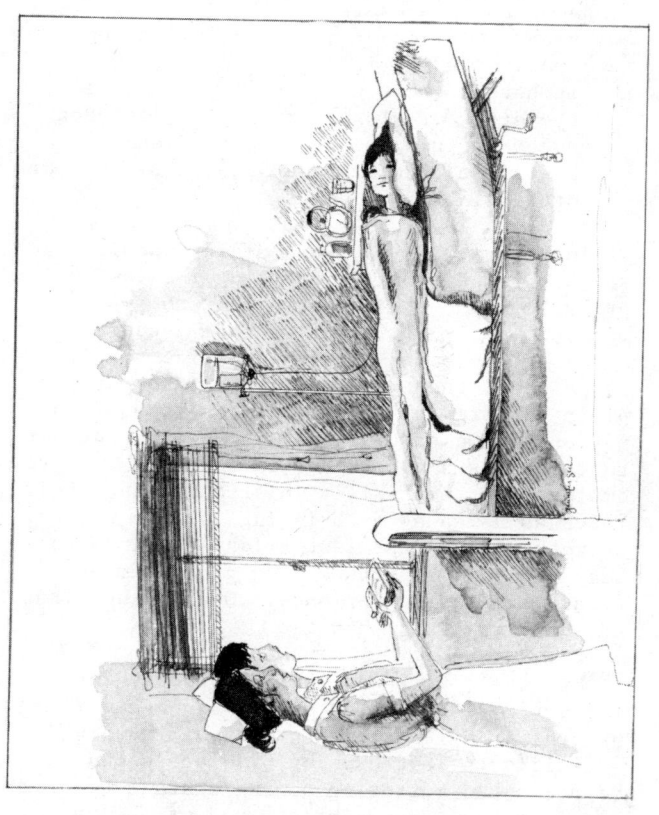

About 80 employees have formed a lay-witnessing club, which meets regularly for mutual encouragement before they divide up and two by two, visit patients and their attendants to give their testimony. They often experience the joy of being God's instruments in a patient's commitment to Christ. One of the members of this group is Tong Chan Lee, and the story of his experience is included here because this is the sort of flesh and blook episode that makes up the fabric of our corporate life.

In February, 1975, we decided to hold a seminar for personal witnessing, basing this primarily upon the membership of the lay-witnessing club. Campus Crusade leaders from Seoul had come to Jeonju, and twice a day, for a week, they had inculcated into our people a concern for the eternal destiny of our patients. On the last day the group went out to the wards and clinics, in teams of two, to employ their new skills in articulating their faith as a means for bringing some to Christ. We gathered, on the last Friday evening, to hear personal reports of the group members regarding their experience. One of the first to speak was Tong Chan Lee.

Mr. Lee's work was that of orderly for the laundry. He collected soiled linen and brought it by cart to the central laundry facilities. That evening his face shown as he recounted mustering up the courage to tell someone about Jesus Christ, and of the response which this witness had occasioned in the patient to whom he was witnessing. Mr. Lee had been speaking but five minutes when from the back of the room someone spoke up.

The Corporate Life-Style of Love

"You've said enough now. It's time to stop."
I thought it rude. Mr. Lee sat down at the
back, then left the room. Then Mr. Suh, an
electrician, explained to us that Mr. Lee's
son, an 11-year-old boy, had just been brought
into the Emergency Room after having been
struck by a truck not more than 300 yards down
the road from the hospital. I rushed down to
the Emergency Room, and found Mr. Lee sobbing
over a stretcher which had been screened off
against a wall. The boy's head had been
crushed by the truck. He was dead.

I was sorely grieved and perplexed. I felt
like saying, "God, do you really know what
you're doing here?" But I put my arm around
this fellow who until a few moments ago had
been exultant in the joy of evangelism and
now as distraught in grief, and prayed with
him for God's comfort, that God would support
his faith through this terrible ordeal, and
that God would receive this child into His
eternal home. And then I went back to the
group to report. After briefly explaining
what had happened and sending the chaplain
down to stand by Mr. Lee, I added simply:
"Life is precarious. We do not know how long
any of us will be here. This gives all the
more urgency to our task of witnessing."

The hospital community rallied around our
friend in sympathy and love. Yet over the
months that followed there remained in the
back of my mind a question as to God's purpose in allowing the child to be killed.
Would his father turn bitter or resentful?
Would he be able to keep his faith in God
while entrusting the loss of his boy to Him?
Much later, I learned that Mr. Lee, who does

not own his own home, had turned over the entire amount of the compensation which the trucking company had awarded him to the Hwasan Presbyterian Church for the construction of a new sanctuary, as a memorial to his child. At this moment a new church is being built on the bluff to the south of our home in Jeonju, an impressive structure that has required tremendous sacrifice from a poor congregation. But the initial gift was Mr. Lee's. And he continues to be active in his witness. He has been transferred to the security section, so that he does not need to collect blood-stained linen. He needs no reminder of that terrible night when his own lad stained the sheets. The victory of his faith is reflected in his enthusiastic smile, a testimony to every member of our hospital community that God gives comfort and power in the experiences of an orderly.

But it was not simply a victory for Tong Chan Lee. It was a victory for our corporate life in that through our mutual support we were able to uphold a member of the family through a personal crisis that became a means for advancing God's kingdom.

These are the events which make a family, a community which shares an ennobling purpose in the midst of duties which may often be humdrum and ordinary. It is imperative to convey to our people that every effort, whether that of the surgical team, or of a laundress, of a technician, or of a dietary worker, is for Christ. He works along with us, companion in drudgery and consultant in crisis, giving meaning to every task, strength for every responsibility, and grace for our relationships with our fellow workers.

The Corporate Life-Style of Love

We live in a glass house. The world watches to see whether we can live in harmony and in love. God has given secular society the right to judge whether we are Christ's true followers on this basis: "By this shall all men know you are my disciples, if you love one another." Our corporate witness is not an intangible thing. Any discourtesy, any departure from strictest honesty, any factional strife, any major argument will soon be discussed in the tea rooms and in the market stalls of Jeonju. To the extent that love thrives in our working community on Dragon Head Ridge,--to that extent we validate our witness to our Lord.

8

O deliver not the soul of thy turtledove unto
    the multitude of the wicked:
    Forget not the congregation of thy poor
    forever.
Have respect unto the covenant:
    For the dark places of the earth are
    full of the habitations of cruelty
O let not the oppressed return ashamed:
    Let the poor and needy praise thy name
Arise, O God, plead thine own cause.

                          A Maskil of Asaph[1]
                          (Psalm 74)

"Does Anyone Know I'm Here?"

Sometimes a few simple facts will jar us out of complacency. Yongjin Township is a district with a population of 14,000 and an area of 45 square kilometers located about 5 km. north of Jeonju. As we began our community health program in this district in 1976 we conducted a survey to obtain base-line information about the level of health in this rural district. We learned that:

> Over 50% of the population is 18-years-old or younger; the average family size is 6.5 persons.
> More than 50% of the women are married by age 18.
> The illiteracy rate is 20%.
> The per capita income is $290 per year.
> Sixty-three percent live in dwellings of one or two rooms, or less than 150 square feet, and 27% live in thatched roof homes.
> Over 57% drew their water from a source contaminated by fecal

discharges.

Over 95% use an open privy.

About 35% have no water drainage system.

Only 5.8% of mothers were delivered in a hospital or clinic, and only 6.9% had any kind of professional help. About 15% of the mothers were unattended when their babies were born.

In the majority of deliveries, unsterile knife or scissors were used to cut the umbilical cord (a practice which often leads to newborn tetanus).

For a delivery sheet, 20% used a sterile or clean cloth or plastic sheet; 29.5% used a straw mat; 28.5% used an empty cement bag.

Nearly half the population makes no effort to visit a physician when sick. Sixty percent state that they cannot save even 20 cents a month for health care.

The statistics are all depressing, but two facts stood out for their starkness: 15% of mothers who delivered alone; and the empty cement bags, the filthy carpets which welcomed so many infants into the world. How often must such women have cried out in pain for the help which never came? For it is not simply the hardship of their lives, nor the suffering they must endure, which must disturb our consciences: it is the fact that they are alone: no one hears their anguish. "Does anyone know that I'm here?"

For most of the eighty years' existence of Jesus Hospital in Jeonju there was no systematic effort on the part of the hospital authorities to reach beyond the gates of the building to the rural communities which surround it. In 1967 a pediatrician named John Wilson came to Presbyterian Medical Center and changed some of our fundamental concepts of health care. It is a chronicle of interest because it illustrates again God's use of historical situations to catalyze new policies, new programs, new blessings. Just as God had prepared Mr. Yongjin Kim, a national business assemblyman, to save our hospital construction in 1970 through kindnesses to his father 30 years before, so God prepared a Dr. Wilson through events that occurred 20 years before.

John had spent his boyhood in Korea. His father was a fabulous character who loved hunting and had started the leprosarium which resulted from Dr. Wiley Forsythe's act of compassion on the Mokpo road. With the outbreak of the Pacific War all missionaries either returned or were deported to their native countries.

When General Douglas MacArthur took possession of Korea for the American occupying forces in 1945 he encountered a chaotic situation regarding public health. All Japanese medical personnel had returned to Japan. Bands of leprosy victims roamed the streets. Epidemic disease was a serious threat. General MacArthur learned that old Dr. R.M. Wilson had worked with leprosy and contacted him in Richmond, asking him to come out as advisor to the military government in the care of persons afflicted with this disease.

"Does Anyone Know I'm Here?"

The elder Dr. Wilson arrived within a week and after looking over the situation recommended to the authorities that he needed an assistant, and further mentioned that he knew a young doctor who was qualified to help. He was referring to his son, John, who at the time was a 1st Lieutenant working in an Army hospital in Camp Crowder, Missouri. John was soon on his way to Korea by troop ship, with about 2,000 in Kwangju. We will continue the narrative in John Wilson's words:

> When we arrived in Korea I was temporarily diverted from working with Dad because of a severe epidemic of cholera which had come to Korea by Chinese junk, and which was concentrated in North Cholla Province. Dave Talmage and I were assigned the job of trying to eradicate the raging epidemic. Dave was assigned the northern half of the province and I was assigned the southern half. Each morning we would get into our jeeps and head for villages where cholera had been reported the day before (this was my introduction to rural outreach work). When we would reach a village where new cases had been reported we would do three things. We would immunize all who would come (and many would come through the line two or three times thinking that if one shot was good two or three would be better. . .). Second, we would meet with the village chief, choose one well as a source of drinking water, and show the chiefs how to chlorinate

that well twice a day. We supplied them with hypochlorite in old beer bottles. Then we would treat those who were sick with I.V. fluids. We would start an I.V. on a comatose patient, ask someone in the household to change bottles when the first bottle was empty, and would leave four or five bottles of fluids, and usually the next morning the patient would be well. We had no drugs, but really didn't need them. Most patients would recover if they could be hydrated. I remember one tragic case where both parents had died with cholera leaving three children ages about 5, 7, and 10. The ten-year-old boy was comatose and the two younger girls were alone in the yard--the neighbors would throw food over the fence to them. I started I.V. fluids on the unconscious boy and told the seven-year-old sister to change fluids when the first bottle was empty--and then give the third and fourth bottles. I never was able to get back to that village and the memory of that scene has haunted me to this day--the unconscious boy lying in the shade of the fence with two little sisters squatting beside him, the bottle of glucose and saline hanging from the fence--with the big sister bravely determined to do her part to save her brother.

By fall the epidemic was under control, but not before 10,000 had died in the province.

When Dad arrived in Korea he had found about 8,000 leprosy patients on Sorokdo Island, with no medical care. . . There were about 1,000 patients in the present Wilson Leprosy Colony, and about an equal number of patients in and around Pusan--the remains of Mr. MacKinsey's colony. These were living in shacks and were mostly beggars. Dad obtained permission to house these in an old Japanese military compound. . . and this became the third colony that we worked with. We had 10,000 patients and very few drugs, and only one Korean doctor who had been obtained to work with us on Sorokdo.

It was during this period that a mother brought her child to see me in Soonchun on a weekend. The child had meningitis. I told the parents that I could get some penicillin from the U.S. Army (penicillin had only been available for three or four years at this time) and that the penicillin would probably save the child. But I made the mistake to go on and mention that meningitis was a very serious disease, and that even with the penicillin the child might die or be brain damaged. With the possibility that the child might become a

'pyungshin' (a Korean term which
includes any form of crippling de-
formity) the parents took the child
home to die--and that was another
factor that haunted me for years.(2)

John never recovered from these haunting
experiences. He carried them through long
years of pediatric practice until the memory
brought him back to Korea. Yet when he returned to Jeonju in 1967 he was dissatisfied
to remain in the hospital waiting for the
sick to be brought to him. He knew that for
the cost of treating one child 100 others
might receive preventive care. He began to
travel with country evangelists, and later
sought to hold clinics in churches which had
been founded by the hospital. Finally it was
decided to seek the government's advice in
adopting a township which might be the object
of a comprehensive rural health outreach. In
those days we did not know the lingo. We did
not know the differences between public and
community health; between primary and secondary care. We did not know what the "health
pyramid" is nor did we contemplate fashioning
a new "health care delivery system." It was
quite simple. We had Dr. John Wilson, a man
who loved children; a quiet fellow who was
hard put to plan a program but excelled at
touching people's hearts; not an armchair
planner, not a theoretician, not a public
speaker, but a doer--self-effacing, low-key,
easy-going, but very compassionate. Within
months the women of Soyang Township knew him.
They would run after the ambulance with their
children because they knew he would stop,
would treat, would take the sick ones into
the hospital. They crowded around him for

immunizations which he scrounged or paid for from his own pocket.

And we, who all these years had properly maintained that the most effective use of a doctor's time is made when he functions in a well-equipped hospital, watched this fellow, John Wilson, with helpless admiration as he destroyed all of our preconceived notions.

And so we came to recognize our responsibility not merely to the patients who come to our door--the critical abdominal emergencies, the acutely injured, the cancer victim, the dehydrated or comatose infant, the jaundiced adult; not merely these, although these are the daily catalog of misery whom God sends to us to receive healing. Beyond them in the country villages and mountain hamlets are thousands more who will never come in, who will wait and may die in their afflictions. What keeps them away?

The three barriers are ignorance, poverty and shame. They are ignorant of the elementary principles of health and sanitation, of the danger of water polluted by fecal wastes, of the communicability of tuberculosis from coughing into their children's faces, of the need to immunize their children from poliomyelitis, measles, smallpox, diphtheria and typhoid. There is poverty. The $290 per capita income in Yongjin Township is far better than that of remoter villages. The vast majority still accept illnesses as did our pioneer forefathers in the American West-- you either lived or you died and you resigned yourself to your fate. They are not willing to come to the hospital because they fear the

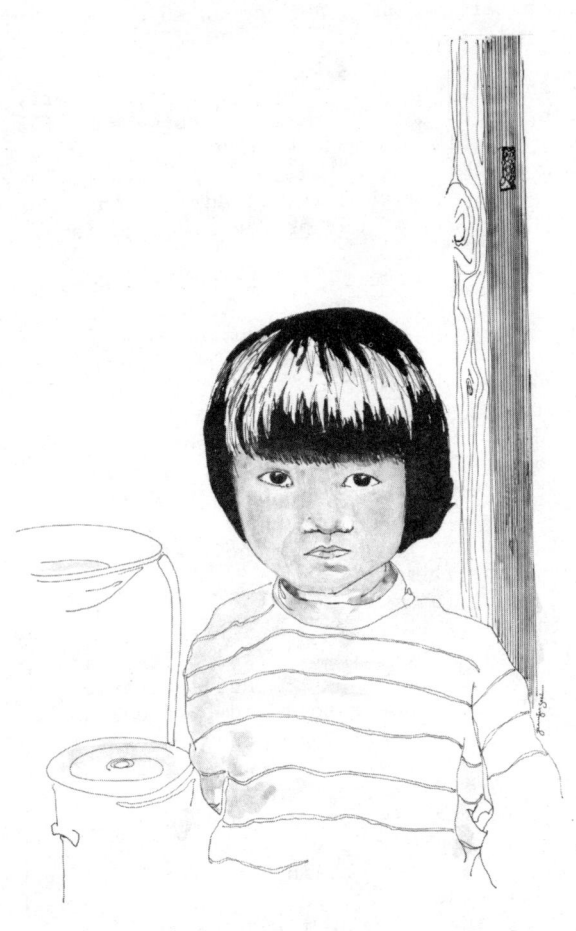

cost, and because they dread the embarrassment. The Koreans are a proud people, and although we have mechanisms at the hospital to deal with the poor, to interview them individually, to refer those who cannot pay to the Social Service Department so that a plan for free or partly free care can be established--they are often too embarrassed. A Korean expression is "I am so ashamed I will die," and this becomes literally a fact. They will stay home and die, afraid to hope, too ashamed to trust in the idea that at Jesus Hospital we will do everything possible to save them, regardless of cost if a life is at stake, never turning away an emergency, always on call to save life.

John Wilson began his work in Soyang Township in 1970. Since that day a comprehensive program of immunization, maternal and child health care, tuberculosis case finding, prenatal and postpartal care, therapeutic clinics, environmental sanitation, evangelism, health education and community organization were carried out. Over a period of six years communicable diseases were virtually eliminated from the area--essentially no more polio children, nor post-measles pneumonia, nor tuberculous meningitis, nor whooping cough; and a profound decrease in the incidence of typhoid fever. The backlog of chronic illnesses was eliminated as the afflicted were brought into the hospital for medical and surgical care. Hundreds of mothers were taught to think about sanitation, were instructed in planning their families, were given basic concepts regarding the care of their children even from before the time of birth.

Out of this experience we have elaborated certain convictions, which I will set forth here as axioms.

Principle One: General hospitals can work in a geographically limited area in cooperation with government health policy and programs, to carry out comprehensive care which radically alters the level of health in such a community with a limited period of time.

Principle Two: Villagers respond with greater cooperation to efforts for the promotion of their health when therapeutic and preventative care is combined than when preventative care only is offered.

Principle Three: In order to promote health care effectively and with a view to long-range continuity, the community must have an indigenous organizational structure established on the basis of grass-roots participation and autonomy.

Principle Four: Community workers can be trained to serve important roles in the health team, and community leaders can be taught to accept increasing responsibility for planning and facilitating health programs.

Principle Five: The medical extension officer most appropriate to Korea is the community-oriented graduate nurse, who works under qualified physicians and with hospital back-up, but is herself the supervisor of aides, village workers and paramedical personnel.

These concepts are not original, but they are basic. They are difficult to put into practice, but they are fundamentally workable. The great intangibles necessary for these principles to be realized are the degree of commitment of the hospital authorities to community health, the caliber of leadership which the hospital can provide for carrying out the task; and the collective attitude of the community in response to the challenge to work together for health. For the venture will never be a squeaky-wheel; it will never adequately compete with the crises which demand a hospital administrator's first priority of time. The men and women sent into the community must have a sense of outrage, of compassionate indignation at the chronic, silent personal and collective disasters which form the fabric of the society they would serve. They must know how to catalyze with perseverance, to exhort with patience, to stimulate without domination. But the ultimate choice is made by the community itself. It must have the freedom to desire or not to desire health; it may choose to hope or not to hope; it may overcome its suspicions and its own internal feuds to seek a better life; or it may prefer to cling to its doubt and its misery.

It is very sobering to be rejected by a community. Love does not always win. Trust is not always triumphant. The venture of a Christian hospital reaching out into a community carries this risk. Ultimately the people must choose: individually, by families, by villages and districts: whether to accept the proferred hand or to ignore it.

But this is the story of the gospel, in fact, the story of both Old and New Testament wherein God speaks to man and requires an answer. It is the theology of choice: the fundamental concept that God requires every man to decide between ultimate options. In a day characterized by the evasion of commitment, the unchanging Jehovah forces man to choose between alternatives which shape his destiny now and forever. Moses standing on Mount Pisgah issued a warning that could be proclaimed in a thousand communities by God's servants today.

> I call heaven and earth to witness
> against you this day, that I have
> set before you life and death,
> blessing and curse; therfore
> choose life.(3)

Our task is to present the options: not only to hear the infant wail, the rasping cough, the birthpangs in the far-off shack, but to care, to come alongside, to strengthen, to love, to relieve, to uplift and to teach: God loves you, Christ died for you. You are precious in his sight. Until that is done there have been no options to choose between, and the question remains rhetorical: "Does anyone know I'm here?"

9

To read the Bible seriously and to open one's eyes to the Chronicle of history is to be awed and terrified. God has declared himself the judge of sinners and his judgments crowd the pages of the Bible and shout at us in every segment of human life. His temporal judgments are seen in individuals and in society and in the whole human race. We see ourselves rushing headlong to destruction--and that no merely to a destruction which is temporal, but to one which is final and eternal. We are given no hope of reprieve so long as we persist in our rebellion against God.

Yet once we have turned to the God of the Bible, to the real God, our terror turns to trust. Because the real God, who has made himself known as Creator of all things, has power and wisdom and love beyond our imagining.

John W. Wenham[1]

Critical Opinions

We must turn briefly to the initial dilemma of this treatise: is the idea of a Christian hospital still viable? We believe that it is. We hold it to be essential to the work of the Church and to the enterprise of the gospel first of all because, when God became man, He healed. There is anguish and pain in this fractured universe. We live in a world which bears the evidence of glorious creative concept, yet is in fact often hostile to the individual creature. So it is of fundamental importance that when the Creator took the creature-form to make the ultimate exhibit of His own character, *He healed*. Christ, who was the effulgence of God's glory and the very stamp of His nature, was moved to remove pain and to restore life and health whenever he encountered those trampled by the abnormal and satanic forces of this planet. God thus is forever disassociated from evil, not merely in doctrine but as a matter of record in human history. This is central to our message. And those who claim the God-Man as their Redeemer and are sent with this message of hope for the trampled, they must heal also. There are hundreds of methods for demonstrating Christ's saving compassion but medical care must be one of them, and the hospital must be one of them; and the hospital can indeed demonstrate God's loving personality tangibly, corporately, experientially.

But the world does not stand still, and our role must relate to social, economic and technologic realities. In medicine, in hospital care especially, the juggernaut of technology rolls on and we are caught up in progress. We become captives to scientific advance. The expansion of technologic knowledge is not simply growing in an exponential manner. Particularly as a result of the cybernetic revolution which began in the late 1940's a process of "horizontal transfer" has come into play, whereby innovation in one field stimulates innovation in another. The mutual feedback creates a three-dimensional growth which is a cone-shaped image rather than a curve on a two-dimensional graph. Think of multiple exponential curves projecting from a given point in different directions along a 360° axis. What is produced is a conical form: the area of a section of this cone at any point along the axis, which is the factor of time, is a measure of the knowledge explosion taking place. The factors that stimulate this knowledge explosion are largely within the technology itself. The mushrooming growth is not primarily a response to the challenge of a need or of a problem. It is more or less self-sustaining and self-propogating.

If we will now bear in mind that this "technetronic" expansion has engulfed the health industry of developed countries, we begin to appreciate their influence upon health care for the world. It is not wholly beneficent influence.

Faramelli mentions five characteristics of the mental posture characteristic of a technological society. These are:

1. *The empirical and pragmatic spirit*, expressed in the idea that whatever works is valid. "The function of a thing, not its essence, is all-important."(2)

2. *Fascination with means*, not ends. How to do something is more important than why, and the result is the idea that what *can* be done *should* be done.

3. *Emphasis upon quantity rather than quality*; not only the notion that economic growth and increased productivity are ultimate criteria, but that only what is mathematically measurable is significant.

4. *The primacy of technical efficiency and economic profit*--the "underlying unifying principle in industrial society."(3)

5. *A manipulative mind set*. Man manipulates the forces of nature in accordance with the mandate in Genesis 1, but he does so employing a purely rational world-view.

When this mind-set shall have captured the health industry we will be subject to a power structure no less fearsome than the "military industrial complex." The heart will have been removed from medical service. Values will

Critical Options

have been sacrificed to efficiency. The sacredness of human life will have been forever compromised. And the trends toward bioscientific manipulation through molecular biology and genetic engineering will have been greatly enhanced.

But the impact of technetronics upon mankind's health is not simply a matter of future speculation, not simply a question for ethical debate in the advanced countries. Because it competes today with the unsophisticated yet basic methods most urgently needed it may constitute a serious obstacle to the provision of health care in developing countries. At the 20th Congress of the International Hospital Federation in 1977, H. B. Richter mentioned three obstacles to realistic care which result when the electronic industry is imported into less developed regions. The *hospital mystique* (the enthusiasm for spectacular cures and the glorification of esoteric equipment) stimulates the appetite for technologic medicine, and in the process further separates people from their real needs. The *quality complex* which claims that "our people deserve nothing but the best" results in care for a privileged fraction of society and neglect of the massive majority. *Sales pressure from biomedical multinationals* is a further hazard. Corporations which cannot identify with poverty and ignorance and malnutrition, corporations which exemplify the technologic mind set, are both unequipped and unmotivated to meet the needs of the Third World countries. (In Brazil several cobalt teletherapy units purchased by the government were never installed because technicians were unavailable. Years later the biomedical salesmen returned saying, "It is for the best because your cobalt equipment is now obsolete and should be replaced with linear accelerators.")

We are thus witnessing an increasing distance between the human predicament and the bioscientific answer. This gap is illustrated by comparing the circumstances of developing nations, in which basic problems remain unanswered, with those of advanced states which extravagantly feed the technocratic explosion. And the gap is daily becoming wider.

The population growth of the world continues at about 2% per year, a doubling time of 38 years. By the year 2014 there will be 8.2 billion people on earth.(4) Overpopulation creates a series of problems, among them urban glut, poverty, unemployment, crime, prostitution and drug abuse.

Urbanization is a problem which deserves special mention because of its relation to medical care. In developing countries the doubling time for cities is 15 years.(5) The number of cities of over 1 million population was 75 in 1960. By the year 2000 over 220 cities will attain that population.(6) In 1920, 28% of the world's population were city dwellers. This figure rose to 41% in 1960 and will reach more than 60% by 2000 A.D.(7) The influx of people from rural areas into cities puts such a strain on food and water supplies, sanitation facilities and schools that cities become uninhabitable.

One of the spin-offs from overpopulation is the decrease in total area of arable land.

The total world supply of arable land is about 3.2 billion hectares.(8) At the present level of productivity 0.4 hectares per person of arable land are needed. Urbanization and conversion of land usage to industrial purposes removes land from productivity. According to one source, by 1985 all arable land will be under cultivation, with an additional 1 billion people on earth.(9) Another authority recognizes that additional land can be reclaimed and placed into productivity but at increasing cost.(10)

At present 10 - 20 million deaths per year can be attributed directly or indirectly to malnutrition.(11) The so-called "Green Revolution" was the cause of much optimism but is now recognized to have been a failure "because the new 'miracle seeds' are only more productive if they are planted in conjunction with optimum levels of irrigation water, chemical fertilizers and pesticides."(12)

There is hope that technologic advances in the areas of synthetic food manufacture, desalinization of sea water, and marine farming will help prevent or delay the exhaustion of food supplies. It was thought that the food needs of the world would exceed food production in 1975, but major starvation in some parts of the world became a reality in 1973, when a drought began which resulted in the death of over 350,000 people in the Sahel region of Africa and caused famine from Indonesia across Asia and Africa all the way to South America.(13) In other words, we have reached the point of diminishing resources already, and the suffering has begun.

Some authorities predict that copper, gold, mercury, silver, tin and zinc will be exhausted by the year 2000.(14) Other authorities insist that substitutes can be found when the price of any of these natural resources becomes too high to make them useful; in other words, through technologic progress. Of one thing we are sure: the reserves of natural gas and petroleum will not last much longer. "The end of the oil age is in sight," says Dr. M. K. Hubbert, an American petroleum geologist. By 1960 all oil discovered by 1974 may have been pumped from the ground. (15)

History will probably recognize that October 1973 was the turning point for mankind. Until that time the Western nations took for granted that technologic progress assured their future. Since that time it has become recognized that we have passed from the "Age of Success" to the "Age of Scarcity." The Yom Kippur War, with the consequent oil embargo, led to a great worldwide recession in the years that followed, but the warning that we are exhausting our oil reserves may have come in time to prevent a far greater disaster from this planet. Coal will help in some countries; solar energy may come later. By the early part of the next century nuclear fusion may become a reality, but not soon enough to prevent terrible hardship in the next 25 years.

The advanced countries consume the most energy per capita. Increasing industrialization produces increasing demand for resources, pushing the system toward its limit--the depletion of the earth's non-renewable resources.

Yet this creates a new set of problems: the dispersion of the unused residue into the air, the soil and the waters of our planet. This is the problem of pollution.

Mercury in ocean fish, lead particles in city air, carbon dioxide in the atmosphere, calcium, sulfate and other chemicals in the water of the Great Lakes in North America; DDT in all land and ocean animals--these are some of the problems we are now seeking to cope with. The most important may be nuclear wastes. The oil shortage has forced Western Europe to increase the role of nuclear reactors in its energy requirements from 2% in 1974 to 9% in 1985.(16) The increase in nuclear generating capacity in the United States will grow from 11 thousand magawatts to 900 thousand magawatts by 2000. The total amount of stored nuclear wastes (the by-products of energy production) will exceed one thousand billion Curies by that year, and 25 million Curies will be released in the air and into cooling water each year.(17)

How much pollution can the earth's natural systems tolerate? By the year 2000 the total population load on the environment will be 10 times its present value. And all this results from the unchecked race to industrialize.

The average industrial growth rate is 7% per year, but the effect of this growth, in addition to depletion of the non-renewable resources, in addition to the pollution it causes, is to widen the economic gap between rich and poor countries. Most of the world's industrial growth is occurring in industrialized countries where population growth is comparatively low. When economic growth and population growth are jointly analyzed the gap in the GNP per capita in 1970 varied from $70 in Nigeria to $3,980 in the U.S. But by the year 2000 the gap in the GNP per capita may vary between $60 in Nigeria and $23,200 in Japan, according to one estimate.(18) In other words, the rich get richer and the poor get poorer.

A sensation was produced in 1972 when the Club of Rome published a small book entitled *The Limits to Growth*. This club or "invisible college" is made up of scientists, educators, economists, industrialists, and national and international civil servants. Beginning in 1968 this international association held a series of meetings which culminated in a decision to embark upon an undertaking called the Project on the Predicament of Mankind. The book referred to is a result of the preliminary studies of this group, carried out at MIT under the direction of Dr. Dennis Meadows.

Briefly, this study examined the five factors described already in this chapter, and ran a series of projections using computers or "models" based upon the exponential curves already in evidence between 1900 and 1970. The factors analyzed were: population growth, decreasing food per capita, depletion of non-renewable resources, pollution, and industrial output per capita. The results of their study indicate that if "no major change in the physical, economic, or social relationships that have historically governed the development of the world system" take place, collapse of the world system before the year 2100 would take place.(19) First a halting of industrial growth due to the exhaustion of world resources would occur, then a depletion of food supplies available, and finally a massive decline of population due to decreased food and medical services.

The gloomy predictions of the Club of Rome in 1972 have been discounted by some futurologists. Some feel that their calculations leave out important factors, such as the use of alternate sources of food and energy, technological breakthroughs in finding new resources and in preventing pollution, and the possibility of arresting the population explosion. It is our urgent hope that marine farming and synthetic food manufacturing may provide a solution to increasing world hunger. We look to research in solar energy and nuclear fusion to compensate for the increasing shortage of fossil fuels, and to avert the danger posed by stored nuclear wastes. Whether the doomsday predictions about collapse of the world system are true or not, it does appear evident that the usually accepted assumptions about growth and prosperity through technology cannot become true for vast segments of mankind. Technology as we see it entrenched to support the Western standard of living today requires such consumption of resources, and produces such levels of pollution, that to contemplate its wordwide application is an exercise in futility. As Meadows and his colleagues put it, there are limits to growth, and if our planet is to avoid catastrophe there must be a "change in values and goals at individual, national and world levels."(20)

Christ may return to preempt this scenario. For many Christians this is not only a scripturally based hope but also an attractive practical solution. But we cannot know God's timing. Of one thing we remain sure: God is Lord of the Ages. God in history calls a people unto Himself, a people whose faith and hope are not in human reason, nor in secular power, nor in scientific technology, but in God. The focal point of history will not be changed by any cataclysmic event which may overtake our planet. The focus of history was the cross of Jesus Christ. The self-disclosure of God in His Son will remain the central fact of the universe whatever else may come. In any event, "Jesus Christ is the same yesterday, today, and forever."(21)

We who have "entrusted our souls to a faithful creator" know that His resources are beyond our imagination, and that His love will never be withdrawn from us or from the world. Others may be dismayed by the portent of socioeconomic collapse on earth. We know that Christ upholds the universe by His dynamic and cohesive force. Others may despair at the limitations of technology. We know that God's resources are unlimited. Modern geology and cosmology are providing information which stretches our conception of God. He is vastly more powerful, vastly more intelligent than we had thought. His love is no less vast.

This powerful, wise, loving God calls us to participate in the unfolding of His sovereign purposes. Participatory discipleship requires radical obedience: we must think in God's perspective, we must pray listening to His voice, we must love at cost. His wisdom must illumine our intellectual choices, His power must energize our wills, His love must consume our passions.

For those of us engaged in medical ministry, clear and sometimes agonizing choices must be made. We have stated that the Christian hospital is a testimony to a truth beyond faith and science, a repository for the concept of human worth, a witness to the supremacy of Christ, an exhibit of a loving life-style. Translating radical obedience to Christ into corporate hospital policy requires alertness in resisting the combined pressures of secular society and the health industry. In the midst of the technetronic explosion and escalating human misery, we must have the courage to opt for human rather than bioscientific values when the options are in conflict. In selecting equipment we must conduct our own cost-benefit analyses guided by the Holy Spirit lest by adding to the hospital cost spiral we deny health care to the poor. In planning measures to heal the wounds of the community we must give justice a greater say than economics. In meeting the crisis of a human soul we must remember how insignificant a few months of survival must be as compared to the vast reaches of eternity.

We are not alone. Every Christian is the church in microcosm, and the church is Christ's body, God's redeeming instrument in the world for as long as the world shall last.

10

Jesus will be in agony even to the end of the world. We must not sleep during that time.

"Dost thou wish that it always cost Me the blood of My humanity, without thy shedding tears?"

Blaise Pascal[1]
1623-1661

Paraklesis

One of my closest colleagues in Korea was our former hospital anesthetist, Elder Tosu Kim. He loved the Lord with his entire life. This devotion was expressed in his prayers, both those he uttered in the operating room before putting a patient to sleep, and those he prayed when called upon at the daily worship services, which in his day were held in our quonset hut chapel. His whole theology spilled out in the inverted syntax of the Korean language:

> Us, who could only die because of sin, forgiving;
> Us, through the merit of the shed blood of Jesus, loving and redeeming, Oh Thou Great God!

Elder Kim had high blood pressure, and one day was brought to the hospital in a deep coma due to intracranial hemorrhage. Half of his body was paralyzed. For weeks he did not respond: and his family and friends despaired. We persevered, however, and he slowly regained consciousness. Months of physio-therapy were required before he could walk. Eventually I was able to take him in my jeep to the Zion Presbyterian Church to attend worship services. We are fellow-elders there.

How well I remember the Sunday morning when communion was to be served. None of us expected him to help in the service, but he hobbled to his feet and came forward to take the trays in shaking hands to distribute to the people. The congregation was seeing a miracle yet fearing a minor catastrophe. But God sustained those hands, and as I stood beside him at the altar, the thought came to me: Should not all of us be trembling, trembling in awesome wonder, as we share the body and the blood of Jesus Christ, our Lord?

> The cup of blessing which we bless,
> is it not participation in the
> blood of Christ?(2)

Dietrich Bonhoeffer wrote from his Nazi concentration camp, "It is not some religious act which makes a Christian what he is but participation in the sufferings of God in the life of the world."

We do not ordinarily think of our Eternal Father as a suffering God. Holy, yes, and omniscient, and all powerful. But suffering? Yet the Scriptures clearly tells us that God in Christ was a man of sorrows, a man who experienced heartbreak, who was perfected through sufferings, who bore our grief without murmur, and who lives forever making intercession for us, yearning for our love. All we can know about the Father we must learn from Jesus, His Son. There is a sense in

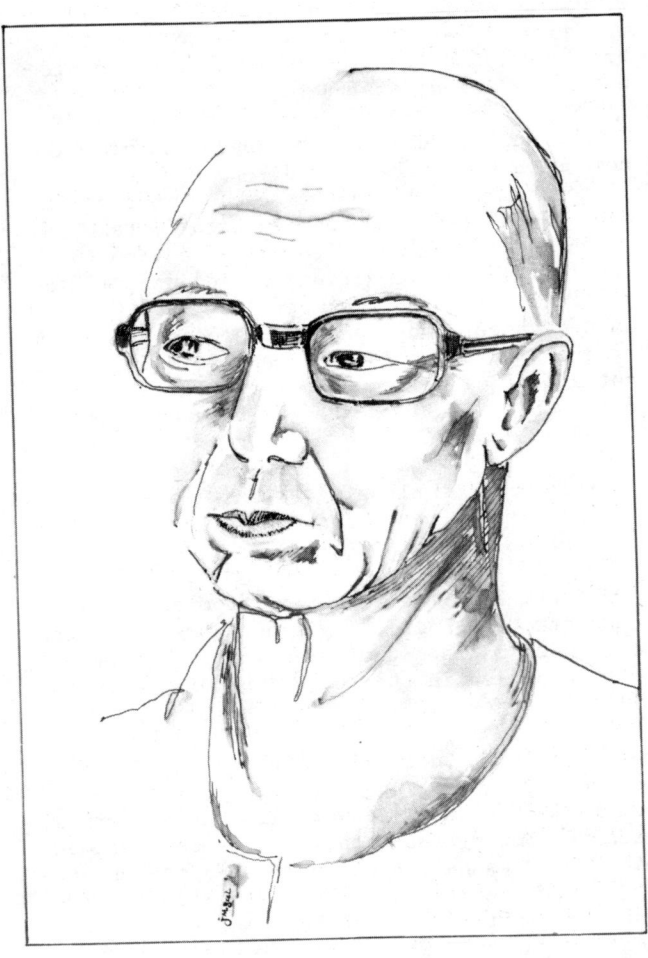

which Christ is crucified in every generation, in fact, every year, every day. God's work in Christ is complete; yet until all men have had the opportunity to accept or reject Him He hangs on the cross saying, "I love you this much."

We believe in a God who touched with the feelings of our infirmities: He became flesh. We believe in a God who is first of all holy: He demonstrated in the flesh that suffering is better than sin. We believe in a God whose mercy toward us is costly; it cost Him His Son. We therefore must not consider it strange if, when Jesus calls us to be His disciples, we find it will involve suffering. The Christian is in fact to be stigmatized, branded for Christ. As the poet expressed it, "He hath branded on such souls His name And he will know them by their scars of flame."(4) Jesus Christ requires that his disciples become instruments to translate God's mercy into the realm of the sufferer's experience.

This was the closing thrust of my previous book, *"Does My Father Know I'm Hurt?"*. Much of the treatise was an answer to the "why" of human suffering, but two challenges were set forth for followers of Jesus. The first of these was the cross of participation, in which we ventured that unless we bear the stigma of Christ, he cannot call us his disciples. The second was the cross of covenant, the idea that the disciple of Jesus must become involved in God's covenant of mercy. In this book we have been more concerned with ministry than with theodicy, more with "how" than with "why." Yet as we conclude we must pursue a theological rationale and spiritual basis for this ministry. Previously we suggested the words "medical testament" to describe our creed of participation in God's mercy covenant.(5) Yet this concept of involvement in God's mercy transcends medicine and every form of health care although the communication of God's message is crippled when there is no healing ministry. God forbid that Christian medicine should cease to be! I am under compulsion to cry out against the secularization of hospitals which were established to exhibit God's compassion. I am constrained to press for meaningful medical witness whether in underprivileged or overprivileged nations. I protest that something precious, uniquely valid, fundamentally essential to the gospel is lost when Christian centers for healing surrender to economic, scientific, or sociopolitical pressures. Nevertheless, I cannot claim that our scriptural directive is exclusively medical. It is surely presumptive to lay claim to healing as a medical prerogative. It would seem wiser to adopt a more inclusive term, to find a more widely applicable doctrine of ministry. Such a concept is found in Paul's Second Letter to the Corinthians, contained in the word *paraklesis*. In the first chapter of this letter Paul sets forth a declaration which might well serve as a charter for medical missions, and beyond that, for every compassionate work undertaken in Christ's name:

> Blessed be the God and Father of our Lord Jesus Christ, the Father of Mercies and God of all comfort, who comforts us in all our afflictions, so that we may be able to comfort those who are in any affliction,

> with the comfort with which we ourselves are comforted by God. For as we share in Christ's sufferings, so through Christ we share in comfort too. If we are afflicted, it is for your comfort and salvation; and if we are comforted, it is for your comfort, which you experience when you patiently endure the same sufferings that we suffer. Our hope for you is unshaken; for we know that as you share in our sufferings, you will also share in our comfort.(6)

At each point when the noun, *comfort*, is employed, we may substitute the original word, *paraklesis*. It is a Greek term which in the strict sense means "called alongside" (*para* = alongside, beside; and *klesis* = to call or bring out). In its usage paraklesis means to come alongside to help; to strengthen, to encourage, to support not in any remote or detached service but by attachment to and involvement in the stress of the afflicted. "*Comfort*" has been given connotations which must be discarded if we are to properly understand its use here. We employ the word "*comfort*" to signify physical well-being, or to express the idea of sentimental though sincere pity. Originally it meant "to give strength" (*cum fortis*). In this sense it measures up to *paraklesis*. A tree is bending in a storm; a beam of wood is propped against it on the lee side to keep it from breaking. A laborer staggers under a load; a fellow-worker runs to share the burden. A man is pinned under wreckage; his neighbors run to lift the weight. Paraklesis means becoming involved in the stress, sharing the pain in order to relieve it.

There are three concepts in this word which need elaboration in order to learn its specific application to medical service; in fact, to any labor of love for Christ. Paraklesis is a godly activity; we cannot grasp it in our own strength. We must always bear in mind that God is the Comforter, God the Sufferer, God the Paraclete.

GOD, THE COMFORTER

"The Father of Mercies and God of all comfort. . . comforts us in our afflictions so that we may be able to comfort those who are in any affliction with the comfort with which we ourselves are comforted by God." No editor today would let a writer use the same word or its derivatives five times in the same sentence. Fortunately Paul's letter was not edited, and the text became a strongly emphasized and reemphasized declaration about paraklesis as both experiential and purposeful.

First, the *experience of* God's comfort is the key to being God's *instrument for* comfort. We can only speak of what we know, the God who comforts us in our afflictions. If I have never felt the need for being strengthened; if there has been no distress or anguish, spiritual or mental or physical, in my life in the course of which I felt my weakness and cried out for help; if in my hour of despair or bewilderment, or perplexity, or fear, or remorse, I did not cast myself upon God and experience His mercy, His comfort, His consolation, then according to this Scripture, I am not in a position to give Christian comfort to anyone else. Qualification for paraklesis is the experience of God's paraklesis. A person who cannot give testimony to what God has done for him can hardly be useful in proclaiming what God can do for others.

Secondly, God's comforting work is purposive. We have received comfort in order that we may be able to comfort. This is an example of the divine mathematics. Those who experience mercy are to become the means of mercy, multiplying the gift. We know that good is contagious, that joy spreads, that love breeds love, that trust creates trust. But this encouraging and uplifting work of our Lord is not only multiplied through us but multiplied for a purpose: "So that as grace extends to more and more people it may increase thanksgiving, to the glory of God."(7)

For a physician to qualify as an instrument of comfort, a substantial lowering of profile would seem to be required. Doctors are adept at becoming tin gods, of clothing themselves proudly in the perquisites of prestige. If this scripture is true, the more they accrue to themselves the trappings of dignity the less able they will be to minister to the anguish of the human soul. To comfort requires the experience of having been comforted, of having been strengthened, a stance which admits of weakness, of common humanity, and of frailty. The first step in paraklesis is humiliation before God. Often the medical profession must regain his membership in the human race from which his sophistication and education may have alienated him. He must not only know his own weaknesses but be grateful

for infirmities which make him dependent upon
God. Every source of human pride, every personal achievement must be set aside. In his
encounter with the sick he must not only
think, "There, but for the grace of God, go
I;" he must be able to say with conviction,
"There, until God's grace and comfort came to
me, I was going." We are but beggars before
the majesty on high, yet we are beggars who
know where to find the Bread of Life.

GOD, THE SUFFERER

As Bonhoeffer has reminded us, God suffers
in the life of the world. It is an anguish
of love and of holiness. It is the pain of a
Father whose children have spurned His love,
and of a righteous Creator watching while His
creation is disfigured. If God could be incensed by the sins of the Jewish nation 2,500
years ago what must be the measure of his anger today! In that day the courts opposed
the righteous, fairness was unknown, truth
fell dead in the streets, justice was outlawed.
Today the courts approve prenatal killing,
presidents practice deceit, truth has become
obsolete, and restraints on sexual immorality
are outlawed. And when every manner of evil
prospers, the Lord sees it, and it displeases
Him that there is no justice; He is outraged
that there is no one to intervene.

God is distressed by human suffering.
King David wrote psalms of praise to the Lord
"who heals all your diseases, who redeems
your life from the Pit."(8) Another psalmist
spoke of the Lord's mercy in saying, "He
gathers the outcasts of Israel, He heals the
brokenhearted and binds up their wounds."(9)

Paraklesis

There is no social or personal misfortune or evil which escapes God's therapeutic concern. He desires justice for the oppressed, food for the hungry, liberty for captives, blind eyes to be opened, the uplifting of those bowed down, and watchcare over sojourners, the widow, the fatherless. If Jesus was moved with compassion when he saw crowds harassed and helpless like sheep without a shepherd, we may imagine the compassion of the Godhead in surveying the starvation of millions, the slaughter of innocent children, the victimization of entire nations by arrogant discrimination.

But God's suffering is primarily related to the abortion of His loving purpose by man's rebellion. It is desperately important to get away from the misconception that human pain or distress is the worst evil. It is desperately important to remember that the fulfillment of God's redemptive purpose for man, collectively and individually, is the highest good. God's love and His holiness cannot be split apart. God loves us in order that we may become worthy of His love. If this transformation requires temporary human anguish in order that man might learn to seek after holiness, or if the experience of trouble is required for my sanctification, so be it. As C. S. Lewis has written,

> The problem of reconciling human suffering with the existence of a God who loves, is only insoluble so long as we attach a trivial meaning to the word 'love', and look on things as if man were the centre of them. Man is not the

centre. God does not exist for the
sake of man. Man does not exist
for his own sake. 'Thou hast created all things, and for thy plea-
sure they are and were created.'
We were made not primarily that we
may love God. . . but that God may
love us, that we may become objects
in which the Divine love may rest
'well pleased.' To ask that God's
love should be content with us as
we are is to ask that God should
cease to be God: because He is
what He is, His love must, in the
nature of things, be impeded and
repelled by certain stains in our
present character, and because He
already loves us He must labour
to make us lovable.(10)

  The suffering of God in the world extends
beyond the first connotation this phrase
brings to our minds. While it is true that
human pain causes Him pain (and this collective human misery must exhaust the compassion
of anyone less than God!), human evil and rebellion cause Him far greater anguish. The
inhumanity of man toward man tears His being
not simply because the "innocent" suffer, not
only because evil triumphs for the moment, but
because through man's rejection of the divine
love God's plan for the glorification of every
human being into lovableness is thwarted. It
is like the agony of human parents when their
children, the epitomy of their dreams and the
object of their sacrifices, turn against them,
and choose lives of shame, hatred, crime,
greed, and desecration. Who can measure God's
anguish?

This is the mankind Christ died to ransom. This is the crown of creation which nailed Him to the cross. And this cross is the suffering in which we are to participate. We cannot add to the great redemptive act of Christ in its atoning effectiveness. The crucifixion is God's unique, costly and gracious means of rescue for every person. But those so rescued must now participate in suffering through the same regenerative process: rejected, slain, raised. To the extent that we share in Christ's suffering may we share in His comfort. Suffering and comfort must be poured from the same cup.

The second qualification for paraklesis, then, is participation in the blood of Christ. If one would truly console, encourage, and strengthen the afflicted, if one would minister to the desperation which lies under the pain, he must feel as God feels, yearn as God yearns, weep as God weeps for a lost humanity: "How often would I have gathered your children together as a hen gathers her brood under her wings, and you would not!"(11)

GOD, THE PARAKLETE

But Paraklesis, we said earlier, is a godly activity. Without denying our technical skills, without disregarding our intellectual tools, without neglecting our scientific judgment, we must nevertheless take fresh cognizance of our weakness, our dependency, and our own experience of being the object of God's grace. A first-hand knowledge of paraklesis is not only essential to our message but humbling to our stance. Further, there must be the voluntary participation in the sufferings of God, His anguish for those in pain, His agony for those who reject Him. There is no love without tears. Finally, there must be surrender to allow God to perform His merciful work.

"I will not leave you orphans. I will not leave you desolate. I will come to you,"(12) Christ promised his followers. He was speaking of the Great Comforter, his own alter-ego, the Holy Spirit. God the Holy Spirit is the ultimate source not only of our comfort but, in possessing us, of the comfort we would render others. He would fill our lives. He would make us capable of thoughts, words, deeds of which we are totally incapable. He would glorify Christ dwelling in us. He would produce in us fruits of love, joy, peace, patience, kindness, goodness, faithfulness, gentleness, self-control--those nine glories which are so far beyond our producing. It is God's work.

We must be crushed grapes before we can become the wine of healing to be poured into the wounds of the world. God will do the crushing, in His own way and in His own time, as Oswald Chambers reminds us. "God can never make us wine if we object to the fingers He uses to crush us with. . . If ever we are going to be made into wine, we will have to be crushed. . . Grapes become wine only when they have been squeezed."(13)

It is for us to submit, to surrender, to be squeezed in the fingers of God, so that He may use us for comfort, the Paraklete coming to the desolate to heal.

During the severe winter drought of 1974-75 the water shortage made it impossible to pump water to the upper floors of our hospital building. During those days a beggar lay in a bed on the sixth floor, covered with wounds and bedsores from neglected burns prior to his admission to the hospital. Because there was no water to bathe him he was sent daily to Physiotherapy, at the basement level, for baths and cleansing. Miss Hisung Koo, our chief physiotherapist, recalls her reaction at first: that it was a waste of time, a waste of physiotherapeutic skills for use in simply bathing this man. Remembering Jesus' example of washing his disciples' feet, and recalling the love of the woman who expended her costly ointment to anoint the Master, the team bathed the poor fellow, cleansed his draining wounds, lovingly cared for him. And in those days the entire staff had been studying bedside evangelism together, so Miss Koo talked at length to this patient about God's love, while washing his bedsores. He accepted Christ as his Saviour. The very next week he developed septicemia and died. And Miss Koo, recounting the experience at chapel, asked, "What is waste?"

Did not God rescue a sinner from the pit into an eternal weight of glory? Will he not clothe him with a body fashioned after Christ's body? Will not that fragment of humanity sing praises before the God of mercy down the far reaches of time? What is waste?

How then did God reach down to this pitiful soul? Was it not necessary to set aside professional prerogative, to humble ourselves before we could comfort? Was it not required to become involved in the draining wounds, to share his pain, to know his face? In ministering to him did we not discover a person amid the bandages, suffering, frightened, grasping at the message of mercy? For the Paraklete came alongside to help, through the tender hands, the pitying eyes, the loving words of three medical disciples of Christ at Jesus Hospital.

Multiply the beggar by five hundred million. Listen to the sobbing from a hundred million huts and hovels in Asia. Think of God's anguished love for those who dwell in the silence of their tears. The Christian hospital may become a beacon of hope to them, but only if it reaches beyond its gates to comfort in the frail and remote shelters of the human race.

Notes

Chapter I

[1] Quoted by Tournier, Paul: *A Doctor's Casebook in the Light of the Bible*, SCM Press Ltd., London, 1969, p. 216.

[2] Ibid, p. 216.

[3] (No reference found, taken from my Bible)

[4] Brown, George Thompson: *Mission to Korea*, Board of World Missions, Presbyterian Church U.S. 1962, p. 63-64.

[5] Ibid, p. 103.

[6] Owen, Mrs. C. C., "The Leper and the Good Samaritan," *The Missionary*, August 1909, p. 408.

[7] The Family Health Care Report: Steps Toward a National Health Strategy for Korea. U.S. Agency for International Development, Seoul 1974, p. A-10.

[8] Position Paper on Health Care and Justice, *Contact 16*, Christian Medical Commission, World Council of Churches, Geneva, August, 1973, p. 3-4.

[9] John 14:12.

Chapter II

[1] Browning, Robert: "Abt Vogler," from *The Complete Poetic and Dramatic Works of Robert Browning*, Cambridge Edition, Houghton Mifflin Company, Boston and New York, 1895.

[2] I Corinthians 9:22.

[3] Wilson, Michael: "The Hospital in Society: Health, Attitudes and Values", *Contact 27*, Christian Medical Commission, World Council of Churches, Geneva, June, 1975, p. 3-4.

[4] Ibid.

[5] Luke 5:13.

[6] Mark 3:5.

[7] Mark 2:9.

[8] John 11:43.

[9] II Peter 1:3-4.

Chapter III

[1] Miller, Calvin: *The Singer*, Inter Varsity Press, Downers Grove, Illinois, 1975, p. 102-103.

Notes

[2] Brown, George Thompson: *Mission to Korea,* Board of World Missions, Presbyterian Church, 1962, p. 70.

[3] Ibid, p. 183-184.

[4] "Health Care: Perspectives on the Church's Responsibility", Division of Corporate and Social Mission, General Assembly Mission Board, Atlanta, 1976.

[5] Romans 8:22.

[6] II Corinthians 4:17.

Chapter IV

[1] Kitwood, T.M.: *What Is Human?* Inter Varsity Press, London, 1970, p. 136-137.

[2] Schaeffer, Francis A.: *Escape From Reason,* Inter Varsity Press, London, 1968, p. 35.

[3] Ibid.

[4] Boethius, Anicius Manlius, quoted in Freemantle, Anne: *The Age of Belief, The Medieval Philosophers,* The New American Library, New York, 1954, p. 70.

[5] Freemantle, Anne: "St. Thomas Aquinas", in op.cit, p. 150.

[6] Schaeffer, Francis A.: *The God Who Is There,* Hodder and Stoughton, London, 1970, p. 12.

[7] Holmes, Arthur F.: *The Idea of a Christian College*, William B. Eerdmans Publishing Co., Grand Rapids, 1975, p. 24-25.

[8] Pascal: *Pensees and Provincial Letters*, The Modern Library, Random House, New York, 1921.

[9] Kepler, Johann, quoted by Hummel, Charles E.: "The Natural Sciences", in *Christ and the Modern Mind*, Inter Varsity Press, Downers Grove, Ill., 1972, p. 234.

[10] Schaeffer, Francis A.: *He is There and He is Not Silent*, Tyndale House, Wheaton, Ill., 1972, p. 68.

[11] Holmes, Arthur F.: *The Idea of a Christian College*, William B. Eerdmans Publishing Co., Grand Rapids, 1975, p. 26.

[12] Psalm 8:4-6.

[13] Holmes, op cit. p. 23.

[14] Hammaskjold, Dag: *Markings*, Alfred A. Knopf, New York, 1965, p. 127.

[15] Lewis, C.S.: *A Grief Observed*, The Seabury Press, New York, 1961, p. 14.

[16] Guinness, Oswald: *The Dust of Death*, Inter Varsity Press, London, 1973, p. 385.

[17] Seel, David John: *Does My Father Know I'm Hurt?* Tyndale House, Wheaton, Ill., 1971, p. 36.

[18] Schaeffer, Francis A.: *He is There and He is Not Silent*, Tyndale House, Wheaton, Ill., 1972, p. 32.

[19] II Corinthians 10:3-5.

Chapter V

[1] Muggeridge, Malcom, quoted in Koop, C. Everett, *The Right to Live; The Right to Die*, Tyndale House, Wheaton, Ill., 1976, p. 80.

[2] Matthew 19:19.

[3] *Readers Digest*, January 1977, p. 55.

[4] Psalm 8:34.

[5] Matthew 10:29-30.

[6] Schaeffer, Francis A.: *The God Who is There*, Hodder and Stoughton, London, 1968, p. 154.

[7] Joshua 24:15.

[8] Lewis, C.S.: *Mere Christianity*, The Macmillan Company, New York, 1960, p. 73.

Chapter VI

[1] Plunkett, Joseph Mary: *The Collected Poems of Joseph Mary Plunkett*, The Talbot Press, Dublin; quoted by G. Preston MacLeod, Exposition, "The Epistle to the Colossians," *The Interpreter's Bible*, Abingdon Press, New York, 1955, Vol. 11, p. 166.

[2] Colossians 1:15-18.

[3] Colossians 2:3.

[4] Holmes, Arthur F.: *The Idea of a Christian College*, Wilham B. Eerdman's Publishing Co., Grand Rapids, 1975, p. 25.

[5] Colossians 1:19-20.

[6] Schaeffer, Francis A.: *True Spirituality*, Tyndale House Publishers, Wheaton, Ill., 1971, p.65.

[7] Ibid, p. 70.

[8] Ibid, p. 65.

[9] John 14:6.

[10] John 10:14.

[11] John 8:31-32.

[12] Hebrews 10:19.

[13] II Corinthians 4:7.

Chapter VII

[1] Lee, Harry, "Madness," from *Masterpieces of Religious Verse*, edited by Morrison, James Dalton, Harper & Brothers Publishers, New York, 1948, p. 404.

[2] John 13:35.

Chapter VIII

[1] Psalm 74:19-22.

[2] Wilson, John: Personal communication.

[3] Deuteronomy 30:19.

Chapter IX

[1] Wenham, John W.: *The Goodness of God*, Inter Varsity Press, London, 1974, p. 174.

[2] Faramelli, Norman J.: *Technethics: Christian Mission in an Age of Technology*, Friendship Press, New York, 1971, p. 32.

[3] Ibid, p. 33

[4] *Readers Digest*, January 1977, p. 55.

[5] Meadows, Donnella H.; Meadows, Dennis L.; Randers, Jorgen; and Behrens III, William W.: *The Limits to Growth*, New American Library, New York, 1972, p. 35.

[6] Twentieth Congress, International Hospital Federation: Discussion Paper, "Health Care in Big Cities," May 1977.

[7] Seaton, Ronald S.; and Seaton, Edith B.: *Here's How: Health Education by Extension*, William Carey Library, Pasadena, California, 1976, p. 5.

[8] Meadows et al, op. cit., p. 60.

[9] Seaton et al, op. cit., p. 4.

[10] Meadows et al, op. cit., p. 60.

[11] Ibid, p. 61

[12] Seaton et al, op. cit., p. 8.

[13] *Chicago Tribune*, October 13-18, 1974.

[14] Meadows et al, op. cit., p. 69.

[15] *National Geographic Magazine*, 145:6:821, June, 1974.

[16] *Time*, May 9, 1977.

[17] Meadows et al, op. cit. p. 81.

[18] Ibid, p. 50.

[19] Ibid, p. 129.

[20] Ibid, p. 198.

[21] Hebrews 13:8.

Chapter X

[1] Pascal, Blaise: *Pensees and Provincial Letters*, The Modern Library, Random House, New York, 1921.

[2] I Corinthians 10:16.

[3] Bonhoeffer, Dietrich: *Letters and Papers from Prison*, Macmillan Company, New York, 1953, p. 223.

[4] Phillips, Stephen: "Grief and God," The Bodley Head, London, 1930.

[5] Seel, David John: *Does My Father Know I'm Hurt?* Tyndale House Publishers, Wheaton, Ill., 1971, p. 63.

[6] II Corinthians 1:3-7.

[7] II Corinthians 4:15.

[8] Psalm 103:3.

[9] Psalm 147:2.

[10] Lewis, C.S.: *The Problem of Pain*, The Macmillan Company, 1962, pp. 47-48.

About the Author

David John Seel is the son of Presbyterian missionaries to Latin America and grew up in Chile and Colombia. After completing his undergraduate medical training at Tuland University in 1948, he served a year in the U.S. Navy and obtained his surgical training at Charity Hospital in New Orleans, and at Memorial-Cloan Kettering Cancer Center in New York. In 1953, Dr. David Seel and his wife Mary were commissioned as missionaries of the Presbyterian Church and were sent to Korea in 1954. They have served at the Presbyterian Medical Center since that time. Dr. Seel became the Director there in 1969 and was involved in the construction of their present 270-bed teaching hospital.